# The Source for Voice D
## Adolescent & Adult

by Sandra Kasper Schwartz

| Disorder | Ages |
|---|---|
| ■ voice | ■ adolescent and adult |

## Evidence-Based Practice

- Of the general population, 29.9% will experience a voice disorder in their lifetime (Roy, Merrill, Gray, & Smith, 2005).

- New advances and techniques are being adapted into clinical practice for the assessment of vocal function (Mehta & Hillman, 2008).

- Data reported in the literature supports the use of voice therapy in the management of patients with both acute and chronic voice disorders (ASHA, 2005).

- Voice therapy contributes to increased treatment efficacy of voice disorders (ASHA, 2005).

- Voice therapy contributes to the cost-effectiveness of medical and surgical treatment outcomes for patients with voice disorders and vocal pathologies (ASHA, 2005).

*The Source for Voice Disorders Adolescent & Adult* incorporates these principles and is also based on expert professional practice.

### References

American Speech-Language-Hearing Association (ASHA). (2005). *The use of voice therapy in the treatment of dysphonia* [Technical Report]. Retrieved March 27, 2009 from www.asha.org/policy

Mehta, D., & Hillman, R. (2008). Voice assessment: Updates on perceptual, acoustic, aerodynamic, and endoscopic imaging methods. *Current Opinions in Otolaryngology and Head Neck Surgery, 16*(3), 211-215.

Roy, N., Merrill, R., Gray, S., & Smith, E. (2005). Voice disorders in the general population: Prevalence, risk factors, and occupational impact. *Laryngoscope, 115*(11), 1988-1995.

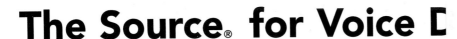

**LinguiSystems**

LinguiSystems, Inc.
3100 4th Avenue
East Moline, IL 61244
800-776-4332

FAX:    800-577-4555
Email:  service@linguisystems.com
Web:    linguisystems.com

Printed in the U.S.A.

ISBN 10: 0-7606-0504-1
ISBN 13: 978-0-7606-0504-2

# ABOUT THE AUTHOR

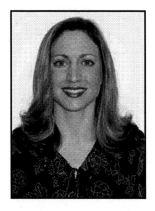

**Sandra (Kasper) Schwartz**, M.S., CCC-SLP, received both her B.S. and M.S. in speech-language pathology from the University of Pittsburgh. Her focus has been in the areas of voice and dysphagia since 1994. Sandy has provided clinical services in acute care, university clinic, and ENT practice settings. She also serves as a clinical consultant to KAY Elemetrics for their voice and swallowing instrumentation, providing videostroboscopy and FEES® training to speech-language pathologists and otolaryngologists.

Sandy is presently employed by the Hospital of the University of Pennsylvania, Department of Otolaryngology as clinical specialist for voice and head-and-neck cancer.

## CONTRIBUTING AUTHOR

**Kelly Teorsky**, M.S., SLP, received her master's degree in speech-language pathology from Duquesne University, Pittsburgh, Pennsylvania. She has specialized in the evaluation and treatment of voice disorders. Kelly is currently providing outpatient services in ENT private practice settings. Kelly is employed by Metropolitan ENT Associates in Pittsburgh.

# SPECIAL THANKS

To Philip Pollice, M.D., who has been a colleague and mentor in the area of voice. Thank you for providing invaluable input and for reviewing this book for accuracy.

Thank you, Joe, for supporting me the past few years, both personally and professionally.

Thanks to my mother, who volunteered her typing skills to assist with this manual.

Page Layout by Denise L. Kelly and Jamie Bellagamba
Illustrations by Margaret Warner
Edited by Barb Truman
Cover Design by Mike Paustian with special thanks to
Blue Tree Publishing for use of anatomical illustrations

# TABLE OF CONTENTS

# INTRODUCTION

The field of speech-language pathology is rapidly evolving into a diverse profession with sub-specialties in many areas of education and rehabilitation. This trend is highlighted by the institution of ASHA's special interest divisions and the current trends toward specialty recognition. Over the past 20 years, there has been a dramatic increase in the involvement of speech-language pathologists (SLPs) in the evaluation and treatment of voice disorders. Collaboration between ENT physicians and SLPs is now the gold standard of care for patients presenting with a wide variety of conditions that may affect the voice.

As this trend develops, many SLPs are obtaining continuing education to gain current knowledge in a rapidly changing field. It is vital that we have a working knowledge of disorders and pathologies that we are now being asked to treat. This "working knowledge" calls upon our ability to incorporate anatomy, neurology, speech science, and voice training.

There are many current texts in the area of evaluation and treatment of voice; however, there are few available resources for treatment ideas and stimulus tasks. Many clinicians are adapting therapy materials and stimuli from motor speech manuals/workbooks to target voice goals.

*The Source for Voice Disorders* was designed to assist clinicians with both the evaluative tools and therapy tasks to provide services to patients with both functional and medical (organic/neurological) diagnoses. It is a functional, clinical manual useful for clinicians with varying degrees of experience with voice disorders

Treating patients with voice disorders may be intimidating for many clinicians, generally because the clinicians treat these patients relatively infrequently. Therefore, this book is organized to provide easy reference of a diagnosis with etiology, physiology, and corresponding recommendations for treatment.

**Chapter 1** serves as a reference to identify anatomic landmarks relative to the larynx and respiratory system and as a review of neurological diagnoses and their effects on voice and speech.

**Chapter 2** focuses on evaluation techniques and development of appropriate goals and treatment plans.

**Chapter 3** covers a multitude of vocal disorders and pathologies. These first three chapters offer diagnostically useful information as well as suggestions for treatment.

**Chapter 4** is a compilation of therapy tasks and stimuli designed for use with patients and can be photocopied for home practice.

**Chapter 5** reviews evaluation and treatment of head and neck cancer patients, including laryngectomy and vocal rehabilitation.

A glossary of terms and a list of resources have also been included for clinical reference as well as a list of references used in the compilation of this book.

The evaluation and treatment of voice disorders is a collaborative process involving many professionals. Keep in mind the medical and social aspects of the disorder to make appropriate referrals and coordinate effective interdisciplinary treatment. These patients offer new challenges to our clinical skills and being an integral part of their rehabilitation can be extremely rewarding.

Sandy

Voice production is comprised of three main components: *respiration* as the driving power or generator for vocal sound, *phonation* as the sound source, and *resonance* to shape or filter the sound. The delicate balance of these parameters determines the overall quality of the voice and will be revisited throughout this book.

This chapter provides a brief overview of voice production from an anatomical and physiological perspective. It is a reference to help you understand structural landmarks, neural intervention, basic laryngeal functions, and vocal physiology. It is important to understand how a change in structure (anatomy) and/or function (physiology) may impact the voice. This knowledge aids in both the accurate diagnosis and generation of appropriate treatment plans for patients with voice disorders.

## Overview of Laryngeal Anatomy (See Figures 1-4, page 7.)

### LARYNGEAL CARTILAGES

The larynx is made up of nine cartilages and the hyoid bone. There are three larger cartilages (thyroid, cricoid, epiglottis) and three paired, smaller cartilages (arytenoids, corniculates, cuneiforms). The larynx is bordered by the hyoid bone superiorly and the cricoid cartilage inferiorly. The hyoid bone provides stability and assists in positioning of the larynx during phonation and swallowing.

### Thyroid

- largest of the laryngeal cartilages
- two laminae joined in midline (approximately 90° angle in males, 120° angle in females)
- superior landmark is the thyroid notch ("Adam's apple")
- protects the internal structures of the larynx
- houses the superior-most cartilage of the laryngotracheal airway

### Cricoid

- shaped like a signet ring
- superior most tracheal cartilage
- articulates with the thyroid cartilage (cricothyroid joint)

### Epiglottis

- leaf-shaped
- attached to the inner surface of the thyroid cartilage at the petiole
- aids in airway protection during swallowing

### Arytenoids (2)

- shaped like pyramids
- mobile joints (sinovial) that articulate with the cricoid cartilage (cricoarytenoid joints)
- serve as posterior attachments for the vocal ligaments
- serve as attachments for the lateral and posterior cricoarytenoid muscles (LCA/PCA)
- serve as attachments for the aryepiglottic folds
    Corniculates (2)—sit on the apex of the arytenoids
    Cuneiforms (2)—embedded within the aryepiglottic folds

The Source for Voice Disorders
Adolescent & Adult

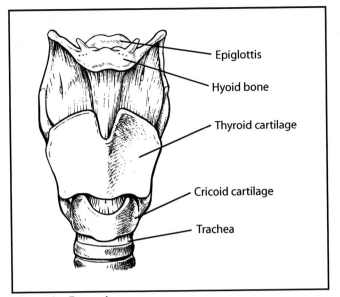

Figure 1. Front view

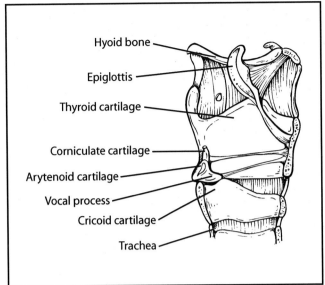

Figure 2. Side view

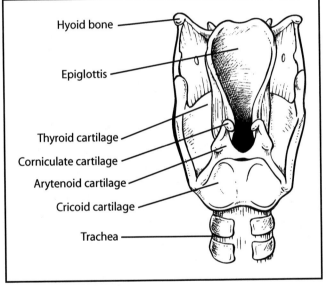

Figure 3. Posterior view

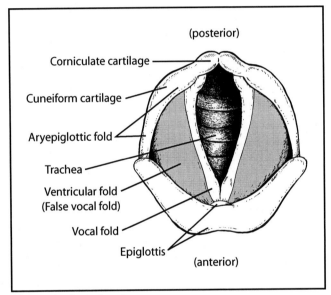

Figure 4. Superior view

Laryngeal Landmarks (as viewed superiorly):

- True Vocal Folds (TVFs)—attachments at the thyroid (anterior) and arytenoids (posterior) (See Figure 18, page 19 for physiology.)
- Glottis—the space between the vocal folds
- Anterior commissure—the anterior point of the glottis
- Posterior commissure—the posterior space between the vocal folds (also called the *interarytenoid space*)
- Vocal Processes—the point of attachment; cartilaginous portion of the vocal folds
- False Vocal Folds (FVFs)—also called the *ventricular folds*
- Aryepiglottic Folds—attachments at the epiglottis (anterior) and arytenoids (posterior); aids in laryngeal valving

## LARYNGEAL MUSCLES

The cartilages (structure) of the larynx are set into dynamic motion (function) through muscular attachments and neural innervation. Pages 8-11 contain reference charts and illustrations of the intrinsic and extrinsic muscles associated with phonation. The illustrations show the locations and attachments of many of these muscles. The charts can be used as a quick reference guide for function and neural innervation.

# Intrinsic Laryngeal Muscles

| Muscle | Function | Innervation |
|---|---|---|
| Cricothyroid | Decreases the distance between the cricoid and thyroid, increasing the distance between the thyroid and arytenoids, and lengthening the vocal folds (VF) | Superior Laryngeal Nerve (SLN)* Cranial nerve (CN) X |
| Posterior Cricoarytenoid (PCA) | Moves the arytenoids posteriorly and laterally over the cricoid, abducting the vocal folds | Recurrent Laryngeal Nerve CN X |
| Transverse Arytenoid | Aids in adduction and compression of the vocal folds | Recurrent Laryngeal Nerve CN X |
| Oblique Arytenoid | Aids in adduction of the vocal folds | Recurrent Laryngeal Nerve CN X |
| Lateral Cricoarytenoid (LCA) | Aids in adduction of the vocal folds; pulls arytenoids anteriorly; shortens the folds while they are adducted; rotates arytenoids medially to press vocal processes together | Recurrent Laryngeal Nerve CN X |
| Vocalis | Pulls vocal processes forward to adduct the vocal folds; increases tension of the folds | Recurrent Laryngeal Nerve CN X |
| Thyroarytenoid | Lateral portion aids in adduction of the folds; shortens the adducted folds | Recurrent Laryngeal Nerve CN X |
| Ventricular Aryepiglottic Thyroepiglottic | Aids in sphincteric closure | Recurrent Laryngeal Nerve CN X |

*SLN only innervates the cricothyroid muscle (serves to raise pitch).

The Source for Voice Disorders
Adolescent & Adult
Copyright © 2004 LinguiSystems, Inc.

# Intrinsic Laryngeal Muscles

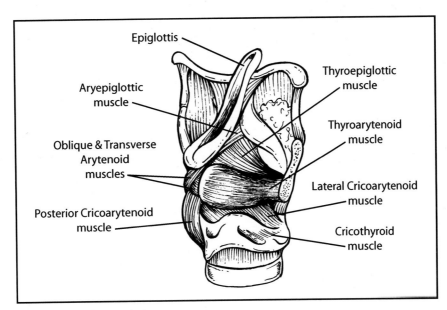

Figure 5. Midsagittal view

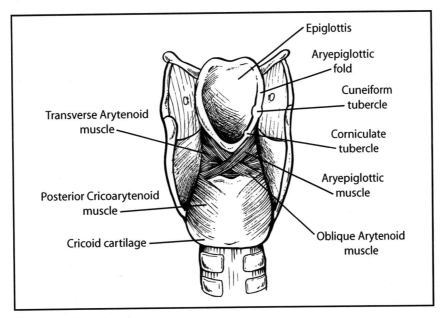

Figure 6. Posterior view

# Extrinsic Laryngeal Muscles

(See page 11 for anatomical illustrations.)

## Suprahyoid

| Muscle | Function | Innervation |
|---|---|---|
| Digastric (major) | Anterior belly: moves hyoid anteriorly and superiorly<br><br>Posterior belly: moves hyoid posteriorly and superiorly<br><br>Both: vertical/superior elevation of hyoid | Anterior: mandibular branch of cranial nerve (CN) V<br><br>Posterior: cervicofacial branch of CN VII |
| Mylohyoid (major) | Moves hyoid anteriorly and superiorly | Mandibular branch of CN V |
| Geniohyoid (minor) | Moves hyoid anteriorly and superiorly | CN XII |
| Stylohyoid (minor) | Moves hyoid posteriorly and superiorly | Cervicofacial branch of CN VII |

## Infrahyoid

| Muscle | Function | Innervation |
|---|---|---|
| Omohyoid (major) | Moves hyoid posteriorly and inferiorly | CN XII (ansa cervicalis branch) |
| Sternohyoid (major) | Moves hyoid inferiorly | CN XII |
| Sternothyroid (minor) | Moves hyoid inferiorly | CN XII |
| Thyrohyoid | Approximates hyoid and the thyroid cartilage | CN XII |

# Extrinsic Laryngeal Muscles

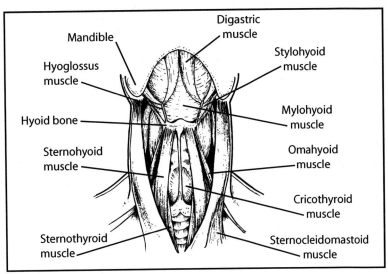

Figure 7. Front view

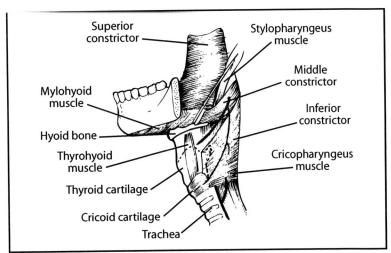

Figure 8. Side view

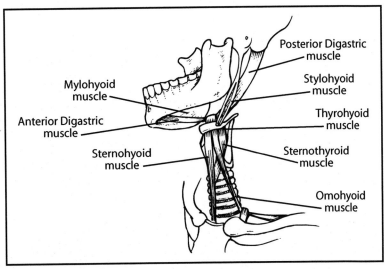

Figure 9. Sagittal view

# Overview of Respiration and Voice Production

The driving force of the voice is the lungs. *Inspiration* is an active process created by contraction of the diaphragm and external intercostals, which enlarges the thorax and lungs. As the lungs enlarge, the air within becomes less dense than the atmosphere and air rushes in (inspiration) to fill the space. (See Figure 10, page 13.)

*Expiration* is largely passive. The passive forces include the elasticity of the lungs, recoil of the viscera, and gravity. As the lungs reduce in size, the air is pushed out (expiration). This airflow may be used for voice production. (See Figure 11, page 13.)

During resting (tidal) breathing, the expiratory phase is slightly longer than the inspiratory phase. Voluntary control of the expiratory muscles extends the expiratory phase and maintains a consistent airflow for voicing.

With the vocal folds in the adducted (closed) position, there is a vibratory "buzz" that can be shaped into speech. When lung volumes are low and therefore expiratory airflow is reduced, the vocal folds adduct more tightly to produce voicing. This type of voicing is described as "pushed phonation" or hyperfunction valving of the larynx. Reduced expiratory airflow may occur because of a physiological cause (e.g., asthma, emphysema) or it may be a functional cause (e.g., speaking in long phrases, poor inspiration prior to speech).

Optimal voice quality occurs at mid-lung volumes and mid-air pressure. The degree of air pressure used in phonation largely determines the volume or intensity of the voice. Normal air pressure required for conversational speech production is 4-5cm/H20. (See pages 28-29 for spirometry measures.)

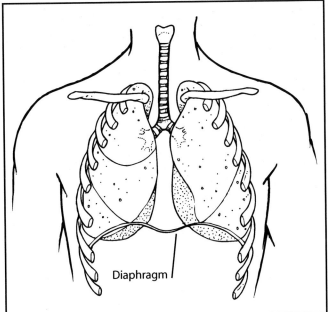

Figure 10. Resting posture

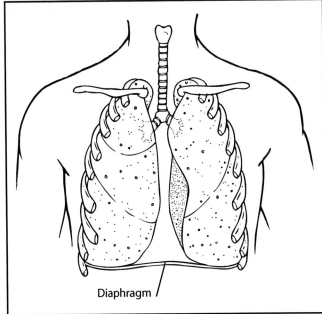

Figure 11. Inspiration

The lungs are covered by the pleural membrane that adheres to the inner wall of the thorax.

The diaphragm is a dome-shaped muscle that separates the thoracic cavity from the abdominal cavity. In its resting position, it is high up within the ribcage. As the diaphragm contracts and flattens, it increases the vertical dimension of the thoracic cavity and also expands the lower ribcage. This expansion causes the lungs to enlarge as inspiration of air takes place.

As shown in Figure 12, there are two paths of inspiration.

1. If air is drawn in through the nostrils, it passes through the nasopharynx, velopharynx, oropharynx, and hypopharynx before passing through the vocal folds of the larynx and entering the trachea and the lungs (and on to the bronchi, bronchioles, and alveolar sacs).

2. If air is drawn in through the mouth, it passes through the oropharynx, hypopharynx, larynx, trachea, and into the lungs.

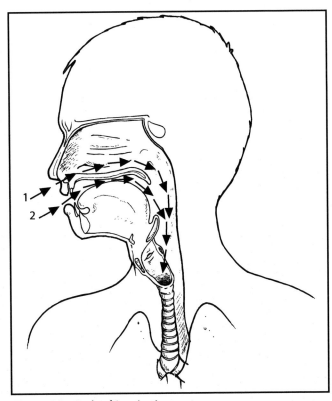

Figure 12. Path of Inspiration

Pages 14 and 15 contain reference charts and illustrations of the inspiratory and expiratory muscles associated with respiration. The illustrations on page 15 show the locations and attachments of many of these muscles. The charts below can be used as a quick reference guide for function and neural innervation.

## Inspiratory Muscles

| Muscle | Function | Innervation |
|---|---|---|
| Diaphragm | Elongates thoracic cavity; primary muscle of inspiration | C3-C5, cervical plexus via phrenic nerve* |
| Internal Intercostals | Elevate ribs | T1-T11 |
| Sternocleidomastoid | Elevates sternum | C2-C4 and spinal portion of cranial nerve XI |
| Scalenes | Elevate ribs 1 and 2 | C2-C8 |
| Pectoralis Major | Elevates sternum | C5-C8, possibly T1 |
| Pectoralis Minor | Elevates ribs 3-5 | C5-C8, possibly T1 |
| Subclavius | Elevates rib 1 | C5 and C6 |
| Serratus Anterior | Lifts and expands ribcage | C5-C7 |
| Trapezius | Braces scapula | C2-C4, spinal portion of cranial XI |
| Latissimus Dorsi | May elevate ribs | C6-C8 |
| Serratus Posterior Superior | Elevates ribs | T2 and T3, possibly T1 and T4 |
| Iliocostals | Cervical: elevate ribs  Thoracic: expand ribs  Lumbar: elevate lower ribs | Spinal nerves at each level |
| Costal elevators | Elevate ribs | C8, T1-T11 |

* the first four cervical nerves form the cervical plexus from which the phrenic nerve branches

## Expiratory Muscles*

| Muscle | Function | Innervation |
|---|---|---|
| External Abdominal Oblique | Lowers ribcage | T8-T12; L1 |
| Internal Abdominal | Lowers ribcage | T7-T12; L1 |
| Transverse Abdominal | Compresses viscera | T7-T12 (maybe L1) |
| Internal Intercostals (lateral and posterior portions) | Lower ribs; brace the ribs with the external intercostals | T1-T11 |
| Rectus Abdominus | Lowers ribs and stabilizes abdominal contents | T7-T12 |
| Serratus Posterior Inferior | Lowers ribs | T9-T12 |

*Exhalation is mostly passive resulting from elastic rebound.

# Muscles of Respiration

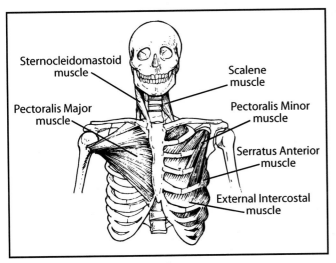

Figure 13.

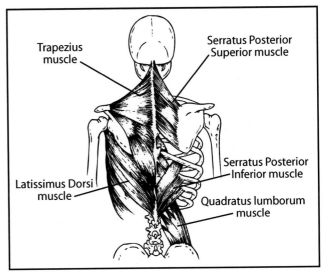

Figure 14.

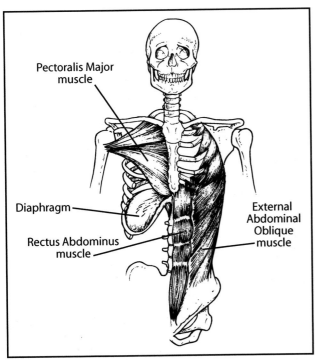

Figure 15.

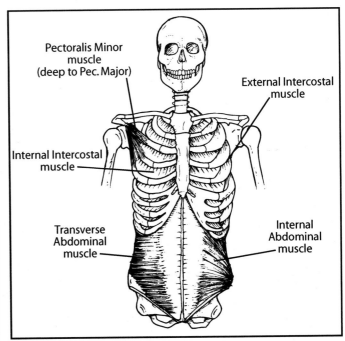

Figure 16.

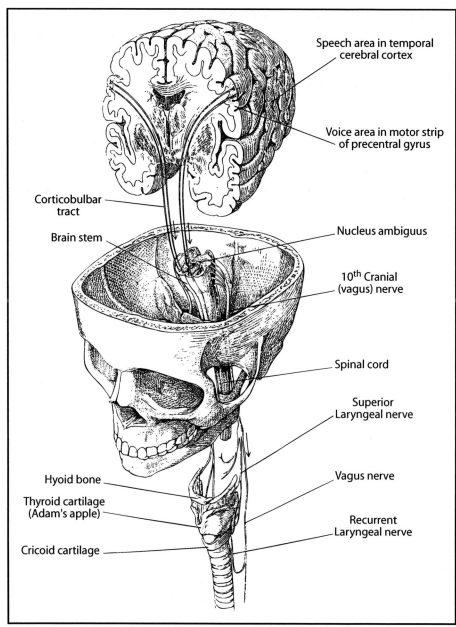

Figure 17.
Reprinted with permission. Sataloff, R.T. *Scientific American*. December 1992.

# Neurologic Control of Voice Production

Speech and motor control of the voice originate in the cerebral cortex. Descending corticobulbar tracts travel to the motor nuclei (nucleus ambigiuus) within the medulla (brain stem). At this point, the cranial nerves leave the brain.

As shown in the chart on page 8, the intrinsic muscles of the larynx are innervated by the vagus (CN X). The recurrent laryngeal nerve (RLN) and the superior laryngeal nerve (SLN) branch from the vagus.

The RLN contains motor fibers (efferent) that control the movement of the vocal folds (abduction and adduction). Bilateral branches of the vagus run between the carotid arteries and the jugular vein. The vagus branches into the RLN with the left branch looping under the aortic arch of the heart and ascending in the tracheo-esophageal groove to the larynx. Damage to the recurrent laryngeal nerve from surgery, trauma, or compression (e.g., tumor) may result in paresis or paralysis of the vocal fold on the affected side. Therefore, if the patient has had a recent carotid surgery (endarterectomy), cardiac bypass surgery (CABG), or esophageal or thyroid surgery, this may pose a risk for damage to the RLN.

The SLN contains both motor (efferent) and sensory (afferent) pathways and branches from the vagus at a much higher level. The motor fibers of the SLN serve to innervate the cricothyroid. Damage to the SLN may result in an inability to raise pitch. The sensory fibers provide sensation to the middle and inferior portions of the pharynx (including the epiglottis) as well as the larynx. Damage to these fibers may also affect swallowing ability.

# Functions of the Larynx

The larynx has three major functions:
- biological
- phonatory
- emotional

## 1. BIOLOGICAL

The larynx is a system of valves comprised of the following structures:

- aryepiglottic folds
- ventricular folds
- thyroarytenoid muscles

The larynx is part of the upper respiratory tract (see Figure 12, page 13). The valves open (abduct) to allow for airflow into the trachea and allow for an unobstructed air supply during breathing.

The primary function of the larynx is protective. The larynx helps prevent foreign material from entering the airway during breathing and swallowing. The valves close (adduct) to protect and additionally can expel air forcefully (cough) to remove the material or irritant.

The laryngeal valves also stabilize the thorax and generate the ability to lift or "bear down." This result is accomplished by pushing air (expulsion) against a tightly adducted laryngeal valve, which increases the subglottic air pressure. This is called the *Valsalva maneuver*.

## 2. PHONATORY

The larynx provides the vibratory power for speech. The tone generated by the vibratory properties of the larynx is shaped by the vocal tract (pharynx, oral cavity, nasal passages) and the articulators (lips, tongue, palate).

Linguistic features such as intonation, vocal stress, and prosody are also functions of the larynx. These parameters help to convey the meaning of a message and reflect the personality of an individual.

Suprasegmental patterns of speech produced at the laryngeal level include loudness, pitch, and resonance. These are complex functions of the larynx largely determined by tension and posture of the larynx as well as airflow through the laryngeal structures.

## 3. EMOTIONAL

The voice can convey physical and emotional states as well. Tension of the larynx and supralaryngeal structures (pharynx, mandible, tongue) can occur during periods of stress, anxiety, or illness. Mood and affective states are often revealed in voice production (tension vs. relaxation). Tension affects the vertical height of the larynx. A tense laryngeal posture is higher up in the vocal tract.

# Overview of Vocal Fold Vibration Theories

Vocal fold vibration is a complex series of events requiring coordination of both respiratory and phonatory events. Inspiration requires the vocal folds to abduct or pull away from midline. The space between the vocal folds (glottis) allows for inspiration of air into the trachea. Phonation occurs as the vocal folds meet at midline (adduct) and air is pushed through them from below or subglottically.

The vibration or "buzzing" produced at the vocal folds is then shaped by the oral and nasal cavities for speech. In order for this vocal tone to be transmitted, it must first be initiated and then maintained. The following theories have been simplified to explain this process.

### THE MYOELASTIC AERODYNAMIC THEORY: VAN DEN BERG (1958)

The initiation or start of the glottal vibratory cycle happens as a result of the following:

- The vocal folds adduct, resulting in medial compression.
- The obstruction created by the vocal folds closing over the airway results in glottal resistance to expired airflow.
- Subglottic air pressure increases below the adducted vocal folds.
- The vocal folds are blown/forced apart to equalize the subglottic and supraglottic pressures.

### BERNOULLI EFFECT

Once the vocal folds are blown apart, a cycle of opening and closing begins, creating vibration. This vibratory cycle is maintained by the following:

- Air is pushed through a constricted space (glottis).
- A vacuum effect is created by lower pressure below and between the vocal folds.
- The suction effect between the vocal folds pulls them toward one another.
- The cycle continues as air continues to be pushed through the space.

### BODY/COVER THEORY: MUCOSAL WAVE

During the vibratory cycle, not only do the vocal folds vibrate, but there is also movement of the surface (cover) of the vocal folds. This traveling of the surface over the body or muscle is called the *mucosal wave*. Mucosal wave propagation has important effects on vocal quality, and its assessment can assist in the diagnosis of vocal disorders and pathologies. First, you must understand the movement as it relates to the physiology of the vocal folds.

The vocal folds are comprised of muscle and mucosa. (See Figure 18, page 19.) The vocalis muscle forms the body of the vocal fold. The mucosal layer or cover is divided into lamina propria and the epithelium. The lamina propria has three layers: deep, intermediate, and superficial (Reinke's space).

This layered structure of the vocal folds, from most dense (deepest layer/body) to least dense (superficial layer/cover), allows for the movement of the cover over the body.

- body: vocalis muscle (most dense)
- transition: intermediate and deep lamina propria
- cover: epithelium and superficial lamina propria (least dense)

The cover slides over the body of the vocal fold during vibration due to these differences in density. As the cover moves, it creates a wave-like motion. The mucosal wave may be affected by changes in the following parameters:

- Length (pitch)
  As the vocal folds lengthen (higher pitch), the cover becomes "tighter" over the body and the movement decreases. On the other hand, the shorter (lower pitch) and more flaccid the cover is over the body, the greater the amplitude of mucosal movement.

- Mass
  If there is increased mass (e.g., swelling, fluid, lesion/mass), the cover becomes tighter over the body, creating a reduced mucosal wave.

- Elasticity
  If the cover becomes stiff (e.g., thickened, harder/fibrotic), it will not vibrate as easily, creating a reduced mucosal wave.

Functional and organic vocal conditions, such as vocal fold nodules or polyps, may have an effect on the above parameters and therefore may affect the mucosal wave and the vibratory characteristics of the voice. These disorders are covered in more detail in Chapter 3, pages 50-84.

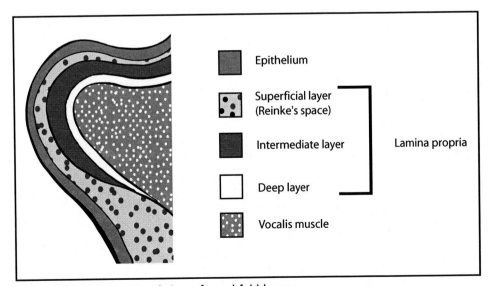

Figure 18. Cross-sectional view of vocal fold layers

# 2 • VOICE EVALUATION

Your role as speech-language pathologist (SLP) in the performance of voice evaluations is multi-faceted and requires integration of both subjective and objective measures. This chapter provides you with evaluation techniques, probes, and normative data to assist in the development of voice evaluation protocols.

## The Voice Team

An interdisciplinary team approach is most effective in dealing with patients with voice disorders as oftentimes there may be concomitant medical, psychological, or social aspects to the disorder (see Chapter 3). Primary members of the team include the SLP and the otolaryngologist (ENT). Secondary members may include any combination of the following members:

primary care physician (PCP)                    neurologist
pulmonary physician and/or respiratory therapist    oncologist
gastroenterologist (GI)                         psychiatrist/psychologist
voice teacher/vocal coach                       social worker

It is critical that the SLP and the ENT collaborate to ensure delivery of both functional therapeutic intervention and medical treatment (if necessary). As the SLP, you are responsible for performing the functional voice evaluation. (Prior to this evaluation, you should obtain a prescription or referral from the patient's ENT and/or PCP.) The involvement of other team members is requested in a case-by-case basis and is often dependent upon information gathered within the case history.

## ENT Evaluation

It is important to obtain a medical evaluation by an ENT physician prior to initiating a vocal treatment program. The purpose of the ENT evaluation is to rule out pathology or medical diagnoses resulting in the presenting voice disorder. Conduct your patient evaluation along with the ENT (collaborative approach) or during separate visits. If you evaluate the patient separately, be sure to request a report of the ENT examination.

A collaborative approach to voice evaluation is optimal for both the patient and the members of the voice team. The ENT often focuses on the *structure* of the larynx and the SLP reports *functional* measures. Since the larynx is a dynamic structure, it requires dynamic vocal assessment combining both structure and function for diagnosis and treatment.

## Case History

The case history should include aspects of the patient's medical and social history. The development of a case history form helps you standardize the information-gathering process across patients. Review of this case history and a patient interview are essential for gathering background information which may prove to be diagnostically useful. (See pages 39-40 for an example of a case history form.)

The Source for Voice Disorders
Adolescent & Adult
Copyright © 2004 LinguiSystems, Inc.

The case history should include questions on the following information:

## MEDICAL HISTORY

1. Review of information regarding any previous evaluation by a PCP and/or ENT, including the reason for referral in order to assess the nature of the presenting problem
2. Review of vocal symptoms and patient complaints
3. Review of other pertinent medical diagnoses (e.g., asthma, allergies, neurologic disease)
4. List of present medications (See page 41 for effects of medication on voice/speech.)
5. History of surgeries to the larynx or recent surgical intubations
6. Family history of medical conditions that may affect the voice (e.g., cancer, neurologic)
7. Report of smoking and alcohol consumption

## SOCIAL HISTORY AND VOCAL NEEDS ASSESSMENT

The following case history items should be included during the patient interview in order to assess the vocal demands of the patient as well as any potential secondary gains associated with the loss of the voice (e.g., time off work, reduced practice schedules):

1. Occupation and job-related voice use
2. Social voice use (e.g., coaching sports, telephone use)
3. Singing and/or formal voice training

# Behavioral Voice Assessment

During a case history review and discussion of symptoms with the patient, it is important to monitor the quality of the patient's voice as well as any associated vocal behaviors (e.g., throat clearing, coughing).

## SUBJECTIVE IMPRESSIONS OF VOCAL QUALITY

Listeners will most often label an abnormal voice as "hoarse" or "raspy." The following glossary of terms (page 22) describes vocal quality more accurately. As a trained clinician, your subjective/ perceptual impressions can prove to be useful diagnostically. Using specific terminology allows you to more accurately describe the "quality" of the voice based on "what you hear" and therefore provides information about the potential movement and/or functioning of the vocal folds. For example, if a patient's vocal quality is predominately "breathy," the inference would be that the vocal folds are not gaining adequate closure during phonation and air is escaping through the glottis.

Although there is not total agreement in the literature regarding the specificity of these terms, the brief list on the next page is for clinical, descriptive use. When reporting assessment results and impressions, use these terms in conjunction with objective measures (e.g., acoustic, aerodynamic) that are discussed on pages 25-33.

## Vocal Quality Terminology

**Dysphonia**: any "abnormal" vocal quality suggesting an interruption of normal production

**Hoarseness**: excessive "noise" in the signal creating an unpleasant, rough vocal quality

**Breathiness**: an audible escape of air or a "weak" vocal tone suggestive of glottal insufficiency

**Harshness**: irregular vocal fold vibrations creating a "raspy" or unmusical tone; a combination of hoarseness and breathiness

**Aphonia**: lacking voice; no true vibratory voicing

**Aphonic break**: a break or interruption in the vibration or phonation

**Pitch breaks**: an interruption in the frequency of vibration of the vocal folds or a shift in vocal register during singing. A voice can break up or down in pitch.

**Tremor**: involuntary variations in pitch and loudness when trying to produce a steady, sustained tone; usually of a CNS origin

**Diplophonia**: the presence of two tones or pitches heard simultaneously during phonation

**Strained-strangled**: perceived strain or pushed vocal quality at the onset of and during phonation

**Glottal attack**: hyperadduction of the vocal folds at the onset of phonation

**Glottal fry**: use of the lowest register during phonation (also called *pulse register*), resulting in an increased closed phase of the vibratory cycle

**Vocal fatigue**: a "tired" voice or feeling of excessive effort to phonate

**Voice deterioration**: reduction of volume or vocal quality with prolonged use

**Vocal tension**: a tightness of the laryngeal musculature during voicing

The terms listed above are used to describe phonatory disorders because they occur at the laryngeal level. Vocal quality disturbances that occur supraglottically, or above the laryngeal level, are often called *resonance disorders* and include the parameters of nasality.

Nasality should be interpreted with caution as there may be an underlying physiological cause related to velar structure and/or functioning (e.g., cleft palate, velopharyngeal incompetence [VPI]). Nasality, nasal emission, and nasal airflow can be measured clinically using instrumentation such as the *Nasometer* (Kay Elemetrics). Assessment of velar closure can be done via endoscopic visualization transnasally to view the velopharyngeal port or via panoramic radiographic/X-ray procedures. Although the assessment of VPI is beyond the scope of this book, the use of descriptive terms relating to nasality is important when providing subjective impressions of resonance.

**Hypernasality**: excessive nasality resulting from increased sound diverted into the nasal airway. Hypernasality may suggest pharyngeal weakness and/or VPI.

**Hyponasality**: insufficient nasality (e.g., denasal voice) resulting from a reduction in nasal resonance. Hyponasality may suggest enlargement of the tonsils/adenoids and/or a nasal obstruction.

## NON-PHONATORY BEHAVIORS

The following terms describe characteristics secondary to voicing that might be observed during behavioral assessment:

**Clavicular breathing**: excessive movement of the chest and shoulders during inspiration

**Stridor**: noise or vibration heard on inhalation

**Throat-clearing/cough**

Quantify any observations using terms such as *mild*, *moderate*, *severe*, *persistent*, and *intermittent*. For example, "Patient X presents with moderate hoarseness with intermittent glottal fry. She was observed to engage in habitual use of clavicular breathing."

## RATING SCALES

Rating scales for evaluation of vocal quality are available in most voice-related textbooks and references to help in quantification and qualification of the degree of vocal aberrance. There is much controversy over the reliability of these scales because of the reliance on perceptual, subjective judgments. Ratings may vary depending upon the experience of the rater (Bassich & Ludlow 1986, Kreiman et al. 1990) as well as the degree of abnormality to the voice (Kreiman et al. 1992). Perceptual training through the use of repeated listening tasks of voice-disordered patients, such as those included with the *Buffalo Voice Profile* (Wilson 1987), is recommended to ensure interjudge and intrajudge reliability.

Examples of available rating scales include the following:

### GRBAS Scale (Hirano 1981)

This scale evaluates dysphonia along the following five parameters (that also make up the acronym for the scale itself):

- grade (degree of abnormality)
- rough
- breathy
- asthenic (weak)
- strained

## Buffalo Voice Profile (Wilson 1987)

This profile assesses the following parameters:

- laryngeal tone
- laryngeal tension
- vocal inflection

- pitch breaks
- diplophonia
- resonance

- nasal emission
- rate
- overall vocal quality

## Consensus Auditory-Perceptual Evaluation of Voice (CAPE-V) (ASHA 2003)

The CAPE-V is a recent collaborative effort of voice professionals and ASHA Special Interest Division 3 (Voice Disorders) to develop guidelines for perceptual voice assessment. It includes the voice characteristics of roughness, breathiness, strain, pitch, and loudness, rating both along a continuum of degree of deviance and whether the paramenter is consistently or inconsistently present. See page 42 for a copy of the protocol. Description, instruction, and scoring considerations are available online. (Retrieved March 2, 2009 from www.asha.org/NR/rdonlyres/C6E5F616-972F-445A-AA40-7936BB49FCE3/0/D3CAPEVprocedures.pdf).

A comparison of ratings using CAPE-V vs. the GRBAS was examined by Karnell et al. (2007). They reported a high degree of agreement in overall clinician ratings between the two scales. The CAPE-V was judged to be more sensitive to small differences in vocal quality.

## Voice Handicap Index (VHI) (Henry Ford Hospital 1997)

In addition to your professional rating of the voice, subjective impressions should also be obtained from the patient to assess her perception of her own vocal quality and degree of handicap. The *VHI* is comprised of a series of questions targeting the patient's perception of her own voice. It is a useful tool to help gain insight into the emotional, physical, and functional components of the voice problem as well as measure therapeutic outcomes. (See page 43 for a copy of this instrument. For scoring guidelines, see table below.)

**Mean values (SD) for VHI subscale and total scale scores as a function of self-perceived severity.**

| Scale | Group | | |
|---|---|---|---|
| | Mild | Moderate | Severe |
| Functional | 10.07 (1.99) | 12.41 (1.38) | 18.30 (1.50) |
| Physical | 15.54 (1.97) | 18.63 (1.37) | 22.78 (1.48) |
| Emotional | 8.08 (2.31) | 13.33 (1.61) | 20.30 (1.74) |
| Total | 33.69 (5.60) | 44.37 (3.88) | 61.39 (4.21) |

An abbreviated VHI has been developed using the 10 questions that are believed to be the most meaningful (statistically) in quantifying a patient's assessment of his voice. This tool, called the VHI-10, takes less time for the patient to complete and is reported to be valid when correlated with the original VHI (Rosen et al. 2004).

# Functional Voice Assessment

Evaluation of vocal function is an important part of providing targeted treatment to patients with voice disorders. After the completion of a thorough case history and behavioral assessment, a functional assessment of the patient's dysphonia should be completed to obtain objective information. (An example of a voice evaluation protocol is included on page 38.) The objective evaluation should include the following tools described in this chapter:

- acoustic and aerodynamic assessment
- examination of oral structures
- visualization of laryngeal structures (if available)

Acoustic and aerodynamic analysis of the human voice is a technical, scientific process. For the purposes of this clinical manual, the basic terms and reference norms are provided to assist in the interpretation of numeric results and how they relate to vocal function.

## ACOUSTIC ANALYSIS

Acoustic analysis of the voice uses instrumentation to analyze properties of a sound wave. It provides measures of frequency (pitch), amplitude (volume), disturbance (perturbation), harmonics, noise, and other parameters related to the function of the vocal tract and larynx. These obtained measurements should be compared with normative data for the patient's age and sex to quantify the dysphonia. Normative data is referenced in the following sections. Instrumentation available for acoustic analysis includes *Visi-Pitch* and *CSL* (Kay Elemetrics) and *Dr. Speech* (Tiger Electronics).

## Frequency

Frequency measures vocal fold vibration or oscillation reported in cycles per second (Hertz/Hz). The perceptual correlate of the frequency of vibration is pitch.

*Fundamental frequency* (Fo) is defined as the lowest frequency or first harmonic of the voice correlating to a physical measure of vocal fold vibration. Fo is determined primarily by the length, tension, and mass of the vocal folds, although subglottal air pressure also plays a role in pitch.

> An increased Fo results from lengthened vocal folds or increased vocal fold tension, resulting in increased subglottal pressure.
>
> A reduced Fo results from shortened vocal folds or reduced vocal fold tension (more lax) resulting in reduced subglottal air pressure by allowing increased airflow through the glottis.

### Adult Speaking Fundamental Frequency (SFo)
(Baken 1987)

|          | Average | Range       |
|----------|---------|-------------|
| Males    | 128 Hz  | 100-150 Hz  |
| Females  | 225 Hz  | 180-250 Hz  |

Male voices have been demonstrated to increase slightly in pitch with aging while female voices drop in pitch (Hollien & Shipp 1972).

## Pitch Range

A reduction in pitch range may be secondary to loss of elasticity or increased mass of the vocal folds. An inability to manipulate pitch may be indicative of superior laryngeal nerve (SLN) damage. Normal pitch range is approximately 2-3 octaves.

|          | Low    | High    |
|----------|--------|---------|
| Males    | 77 Hz  | 576 Hz  |
| Females  | 134 Hz | 895 Hz  |

*(Baken 1987)*

## Amplitude/Intensity

Intensity is also called *energy* and measures the amplitude or vertical magnitude of the sound waveform. The perceptual correlate of amplitude is volume or loudness reported in decibels (dB).

In order to raise volume or increase intensity, the vocal folds are medially compressed, offering increased glottal resistance to airflow. This action creates an increase in subglottal air pressure. (See measures, page 30.) Average conversational speech is 70-80dB sound pressure level (SPL).

|          | Mean    |
|----------|---------|
| Males    | 77.8 dB |
| Females  | 74.0 dB |

*(Holmberg et al. 1994)*

Note: SPL can also be measured independently from acoustics using a sound level meter, which is an instrument measuring the intensity of a sound in dB.

## Perturbation

Perturbation refers to a disturbance in the regularity of the waveform. These disturbances reflect slight changes in the mass, tension, or vibratory characteristics of the vocal folds from one glottic cycle to the next. Perturbation correlates to perceived roughness or harshness.

Instrumental acoustic analysis of pitch and volume during sustained vowel production of /a/ often includes reported measurements of perturbation. An increase in perturbation measures is perceived as hoarseness. Although there is some degree of perturbation in normal voices, there is an increased percent in dysphonic voices.

Clinicians should be cautious in the interpretation of perturbation measure as the type of waveform (signal) varies dependent upon the distortion or aperiodicity of the signal (Titze 1995). Perturbation also varies as a function of pitch. As a result, there is a wide range of "norms" reported in the literature. General definitions and examples of the most frequently reported clinical reference norms and their sources are listed below. Values above these normative measures are seen in dysphonic patients.

**Jitter** is a short-term measure of cycle-to-cycle variation in fundamental frequency detected during a sustained vowel. Jitter is considered a measure of instability from cycle to cycle in the vibratory characteristics of the vocal folds. Average jitter is expressed as a percent of the average fundamental frequency with normal perturbation (variation from cycle to cycle) reported to be less than one percent. Mean absolute jitter represents pitch variations occurring between consecutive pitch periods and is expressed in microseconds.

Jitter % = < 1.0%

Mean absolute jitter = 0.4msec

**Shimmer** is a short-term measure of cycle-to-cycle variation in amplitude detected during a sustained vowel. Shimmer reflects slight changes or irregularity in intensity of the signal. The norm is reported as less than 0.5 dB variation from cycle to cycle and/or less than 5 percent of the average amplitude.

Shimmer in dB = < 0.5 dB

Shimmer percent = < 5 %

**Harmonics-to-Noise Ratio (H/N)** is also called signal-to-noise ratio and is a measure of the frequency structure (harmonics) of the voice signal to the noise within that signal. Increased noise in a speech signal results in a lower H/N ratio and is perceived as hoarseness. Therefore, for this measure, any value below the reported norm is seen in dysphonic patients. The norm for harmonics-to-noise may be expressed as a ratio or in decibels. Normative values are greater than 1.0 or greater than 12dB (meaning that the harmonic energy is greater than the energy from noise).

**Harmonics** are defined as multiples of the fundamental frequency.

**Noise** is defined as aperiodic or random distribution of acoustical energy.

H/N = >12dB

**Additional Tasks Recommended During Instrumental Acoustic Analysis**

The following tasks are recommendations adapted from Titze (1995):

- An audio recording of the patient's voice using a professional grade microphone is recommended for a baseline and post-treatment comparison, as well as to make perceptual judgments regarding vocal quality. Set the microphone at a constant microphone-to-mouth distance (approximately three to four centimeters at a 45-90 degree angle from the mouth. Record both a conversational and a reading sample.

  The "Rainbow Passage" is frequently used for this sample. (See page 44.)

- Acoustic analysis of pitch and amplitude during automatic speech tasks (e.g., counting) and sentence production.

  Instruct the patient to say the following sentences:

  "Where are you going?" (recommended for assessment of continuous voicing since the sentence contains only voiced consonants)

  "The blue spot is on the key again." (recommended for assessment of voiced and voiceless onsets)

## AERODYNAMIC ASSESSMENT

## Airflow Measurement

Measurements of airflow are important as vocal fold vibration is activated and maintained by respiratory drive. (See Chapter 1, page 18.) Devices used to measure aerodynamics during speech include the *Aerophone* (Kay Elemetrics) and *Phonatory Function Analyzer* (Nagashima).

If the patient has been seen by a pulmonary (lung) specialist and has undergone pulmonary evaluation or Pulmonary Function Testing (PFT) prior to his referral for voice assessment, request a copy of these results. This testing will provide you with measures of respiratory function.

### Spirometry

When available, spirometry is used to assess lung volume and capacity. Spirometry measures volume displacement of air or water during inhalatory and exhalatory tasks and is measured in cubic centimeters (cc) or liters (L). Spirometry is a non-invasive measure obtained as the patient breathes into a tube placed in the mouth. The instrument measures displacement of water (wet spirometry) or air (dry spirometry) through closed chambers during expiratory tasks. The resulting changes in volume provide information about the volume of air moved by the patient.

Terms and norms used in spirometry are as follows:

**Tidal volume** (TV) is the volume of air inspired and expired (moved) during a typical resting respiratory cycle (750cc).

**Inspiratory reserve volume** (IRV) is the volume of air that can be inspired after normal tidal inspiration (1500-2500cc).

**Expiratory reserve volume** (ERV) is the maximum volume that can be expired beyond spontaneous or tidal expiration (1500-2000cc).

**Residual volume** (RV) is the volume of gas/air remaining in the lungs after maximum expiration; the residual lung volume that cannot be expelled (1000-1500cc).

**Vital capacity** (VC) is the total volume of air that can expired after maximal inhalation (3500-5000cc for normal healthy males). VC is affected by height, weight, and age.

## Glottal Airflow

Measurements of subglottal and transglottal airflow are important in the assessment of vocal efficiency. As discussed in Chapter 1, vocal fold vibration is initiated and maintained by subglottic pressure that is greater than supraglottic pressure in order to push air through the glottis. Comparison of what is happening at the subglottis (pressure) and supraglottis (flow) allows us to determine what is happening at the glottis or level of the vocal folds. Aerodynamic measures that are considered to be within normal limits (WNL) suggest normal or efficient functioning of the vocal folds.

Abnormally high subglottic pressure and glottal resistance may be indicative of vocal hyperfunction or increased mass, whereas increased glottal airflow may be seen in cases of poor adduction, such as presbylarynx or vocal fold paralysis. Airflow measures are useful in clinical practice when comparing pre- and post-results of medical, surgical, or therapeutic intervention.

Note: Airflow measures are known to be variable across repeated trials, even in normal subjects, secondary to the physical effort the patient exerts as well as practice effects across multiple trials. An average of two trials is often reported.

The most commonly obtained and reported aerodynamic measures in clinical practice are the following:
- air pressure
- airflow
- glottal resistance

*Air Pressure*

Air pressure is measured either directly or indirectly and results are reported in cmH2O (centimeters of water).

Direct measurement involves the insertion of a hypodermic needle into the cricothyroid space that is connected to a pressure transducer measuring pressure below the adducted vocal folds.

Indirect measurement is the most common method, involving a tube placed intraorally that measures the pressure behind the lips just prior to opening during plosive productions (e.g., /p/). The intraoral pressure generated behind the lips is highly correlated to subglottic pressure or pressure below the adducted vocal folds (Smitheran & Hixon 1981).

### Subglottic Pressure (cmH20)
(Holmberg et al. 1994)

|  | Mean | Standard Deviation |
|---|---|---|
| Males | 5.9 | 1.0 |
| Females | 5.5 | 1.2 |

Within normal limits (WNL) is often reported as a patient's ability to maintain 5cmH20 for 5 seconds (Netsell & Hixon 1978).

*Airflow*

Instrumental measurement of airflow involves the use of a mouthpiece or face mask in place during sustained vowel production, therefore maintaining an open vocal tract. The unit of measure is volume of air displaced per unit of time (liters/second [L/s]).

Average airflow is reported as 100-200cc/sec with the following differences between males and females expressed in liters per second (L/s) (Holmberg et al. 1994).

### Airflow (L/s)

|  | Mean | Standard Deviation |
|---|---|---|
| Males | 0.2 | 0.06 |
| Females | 0.2 | 0.08 |

*Glottal Resistance*

Glottal resistance is measured by obtaining the ratio between the average subglottic air pressure and the average glottal airflow (pressure/flow = cmH20/L/sec). Differences between males and females is reported as follows (Holmberg et al. 1994):

### Glottal Resistance (cm H20/L/sec)

|         | Mean | Standard Deviation |
|---------|------|--------------------|
| Males   | 32.6 | 13.7               |
| Females | 30.8 | 9.4                |

## Measures of Vibratory Cycle:  Glottal Waveform Analysis

Glottal waveform analysis provides information regarding the degree of opening and closing of the vocal folds during a vibratory cycle. Although these measures have historically been reported in the research literature only, they are becoming more commonly used in clinical assessment. Publications reporting quantification measures of Electroglottograph (EGG) waveforms in normal subjects include Higgins et al. 1994 and Baken & Orlikoff 1999.

Two methods in which glottal waveforms are represented and analyzed include EGG and inverse filtering.

### EGG

EGG produces a visual representation (waveform) of the ratio of open phase to closed phase during the glottic cycle and therefore is used as a technique to assess vocal fold contact.

EGG waveform (Lx) is obtained by using two small electrodes placed on opposite sides of the neck at the level of the vocal folds (on each thyroid laminae). A weak electrical current is passed from one electrode to the other, responding to changes in impedance created by vocal fold contact during vibration. This electrical current is then translated into a waveform, using an oscillograph for visual display.

Normal EGG representation displays:  (labeled "abc" in Figure 19)
- sharp rise to indicate closing of the vocal folds (a)
- sloping return to indicate opening of the vocal folds (b)
- baseline signal occurs during the open phase of vibration (c)

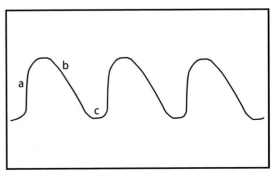

Figure 19.  Normal

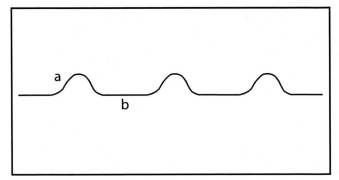

Figure 20. Breathy

A breathy voice would display a gradual rise as the vocal folds close (a) and an excessively long open phase (b). (Conversely, a pressed or strained voice would result from an increased duration of the closed phase of vibration.)

Aperiodic vocal fold vibration in dysphonic voices is displayed visually as asymmetry from one cycle to the next.

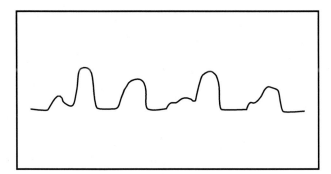

Figure 21. Aperiodic

## Inverse Filtering

Using a mask, inverse filtering records oral airflow and "filters out" the resonant properties of the supraglottic cavities. The result, called a *flow glottogram*, is an estimated waveform produced at the vocal folds during sustained vowel production. This waveform is often used as a complement to EGG to measure airflow in comparison with glottal closure patterns.

The representation of the flow glottogram waveform displays:
- peak during glottal airflow (open phase) (a)
- trough during vocal fold contact (closed phase) (b)

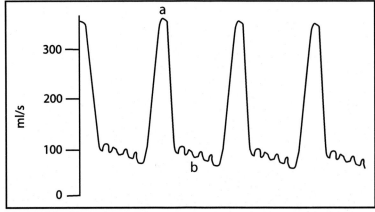

Figure 22. Flow glottogram

The resulting measures of glottal waveform assessment most often reported in clinical assessment/report writing include open quotient and speed quotient. *Open quotient* represents the duration of the open phase in relation to the duration of the entire glottal cycle. The norm for this measure is 0.5 (Titze 1994), meaning that the open phase is approximately half as long as the entire cycle.

Open Quotient: $\dfrac{\text{duration of the open phase}}{\text{duration of the entire cycle}}$

norm = 0.5

The speed quotient represents the speed with which the vocal folds open versus close. The norm is reported (Titze 1994) as 1.0, meaning the speed of opening to closing when compared should be relatively equal to each other.

Speed Quotient: $\dfrac{\text{average speed of opening}}{\text{average speed of closing}}$

norm = 1.0

## Non-Instrumental Assessment

You may not have access to acoustic and aerodynamic assessment instrumentation within your practice setting. Although the following non-instrumental assessment techniques offer less precise measurements of vocal function, they do provide information regarding respiratory and laryngeal functioning.

- pitch range
- maximum phonation time (MPT)

- *s/z* ratio
- speaking rate

### PITCH RANGE

Measures of pitch range are used to assess vocal flexibility and SLN function (may also be measured objectively during acoustic analysis, page 26).

Instruct the patient to start at his lowest possible note/pitch and produce vocal tones upward in pitch. (Use a pitch pipe or keyboard, if needed.) Count the notes from the bottom of the patient's pitch range to the top. The norm is two to three octaves.

### MAXIMUM PHONATION TIME (MPT)

MPT is an estimated measure of airflow during voicing.

Instruct the patient to sustain the vowel /a/ at a comfortable pitch and loudness on a single breath until he "runs out of air." This measure is related to air expenditure and may vary on multiple trials. An average of three trials is recommended. The norm is 15-20 seconds. Reduced MPT may suggest poor respiratory support or poor medial glottal closure.

## S/Z RATIO

S/Z ratio is a comparative measure of sustained voiceless/voiced cognate pair productions (Eckel & Boone 1981).

Time the patient as she sustains a /s/ as long as possible on a single breath. Then do the same for a sustained /z/. Use two trials and vary the order, taking the longest of the two productions. The expected ratio of production times should be 1:1 reflecting equal duration of airflow for each production regardless of the voiceless or voiced parameter. A ratio of greater than 1:4 suggests vibratory dysfunction of the vocal folds, possible laryngeal pathology, glottal inefficiency, or excessive compression at the laryngeal level.

## SPEAKING RATE

Speaking rate may be assessed during speaking or reading and is reported in either words per minute (WPM) or syllables per minute (SPM). These measures and observation of breath patterns and phrasing lengths a speaker is using will help in your assessment of respiratory functioning. Poor respiratory functioning may result in the use of short phrases and reduced rate (need for more frequent breaths).

Normal speaking rates for adults:
115-165 WPM or 162-230 SPM (Andrews & Ingham 1971)

Normal reading rates for adults:
210-265 SPM (Peters & Guitar 1991)

# Vocal Tract Visualization

The vocal tract may be visualized by either direct or indirect examination and conducted by either an ENT physician or a trained SLP. Official documents published by ASHA (2004) provide professional guidelines for the performance of laryngeal examinations by SLPs.

The most common methods used in clinical practice to visualize laryngeal structures are described on the next page, including the benefits and disadvantages of each method. The method for visualization performed is often dependent upon the instrumentation available to the examiner (ENT/SLP) in his/her practice setting, as well as the examiner's level of training with each procedure.

## INDIRECT VISUALIZATION (use of laryngeal mirror intraorally)

| Advantages | Disadvantages |
| --- | --- |
| inexpensive | information not archived for review |
| easy to use | unable to view running speech |
| quick to administer | may elicit gag reflex |
| easy to disinfect the mirror | |

## DIRECT VISUALIZATION

### Fiberoptic laryngoscopy (FOL) or naso-pharyngeal laryngoscopy (NPL)
(use of a fiberoptic endoscope transnasally)

**Advantages**
excellent visualization of larynx
able to view velopharynx
able to archive image for review
able to visualize running speech
bypasses gag reflex

**Disadvantages**
expensive
uncomfortable for patient

### Rigid laryngoscopy
(use of a rigid telescope transorally; the angle of the scope may be 70 or 90 degrees)

**Advantages**
high illumination of structures
excellent image quality
wide field of view
able to archive for review

**Disadvantages**
expensive
may elicit gag reflex
unable to view running speech

### Other assessment tools

High speed video is another tool used for laryngeal visualization. High speed video records images at a higher rate, allowing more frames of visualization per second. It is useful for obtaining views of brief voicing events such as voice onset, spasms, and vocal fold vibrations that are irregular (aperiodic).

Laryngeal ultrasound is a technique which is currently being investigated in terms of its ability to assess laryngeal structure and identify laryngeal pathology.

Laryngeal EMG (electromyography) is a test performed by an ENT or neurologist to study laryngeal muscle activities under various conditions. This technique is often used to assist with the diagnosis of conditions such as vocal fold paralysis (page 59) or spasmodic dysphonia (page 61).

Although these laryngeal assessment procedures are not yet standard in most practices or used routinely for clinical diagnosis, they are increasingly being used and reported in literature as alternative techniques for evaluating the larynx.

## VIDEOLARYNGEALSTROBOSCOPY (VLS)

### Basics
Use of stroboscopy during laryngeal examination represents state of the art visualization. It uses either flexible or rigid endoscopy combined with a stroboscopic light that emits timed flashes asynchronized with the frequency of vocal fold vibration. The result is apparent slow motion because each successive flash illuminates a different phase of the vibratory cycle, revealing an average pattern of vibration across multiple cycles.

Stroboscopy allows visualization of vocal fold vibratory patterns demonstrated to be diagnostically useful in the evaluation and treatment of patients with voice disorders (Bless et al. 1987, Sataloff et al. 1988, Woo et al. 1991).

## Interpretation

As discussed in Chapter 1, changes in length, mass, and stiffness of the vocal folds result in vibratory changes that have qualitative effects on the voice. Assessments of these vibratory characteristics are made through perceptual judgments by trained SLPs. A thorough understanding of laryngeal anatomy and vocal fold physiology is essential as well as knowledge of how the vibratory properties of the vocal folds vary respective to changes in frequency and intensity. Special training and continuing education is recommended to become competent in the interpretation of laryngeal functioning as seen on videostroboscopy (ASHA 2004). See page 45 for an example of a consent form used for performance of videostroboscopy. Example protocol for videostroboscopy examination can be found on page 46.

## Parameters

The following parameters have become standard practice in the interpretation of stroboscopic laryngeal images (Bless et al. 1987). You can assess these parameters under stroboscopic examination while the patient is phonating at a comfortable pitch and loudness. Use phonatory tasks of increasing and decreasing pitch and loudness to record changes observed in these parameters.

**Symmetry**—the degree that the vocal folds provide mirror images of one another

**Glottic closure**—the degree that the vocal folds approximate during the closed phase of vibration

**Amplitude**—the extent of horizontal excursion of the vocal folds during movement

**Periodicity**—the regularity of successive cycles of vibration

**Mucosal wave**—the mucosa traveling over the body of the vocal fold from the medial edge to two-thirds the width of the true vocal fold (traveling laterally)

**Hyperfunction**—increased supraglottic tension or the presence of false fold adduction

## Benefits

The use of stroboscopy during laryngeal examination has the following benefits:
- allows for assessment of vibration and mucosal wave
- aids in differential diagnoses of organic pathologies
- aids in functional diagnoses
- allows for a frame-by-frame analysis

- provides documentation of laryngeal structures (e.g., video, hard copy photos)
- increases patient's understanding of laryngeal functioning and/or pathology
- provides biofeedback for the patient to gain visual representation of laryngeal movements during voice production

# Clinical Report Writing

It is important to remember that only a physician can render a medical diagnosis. Your role as SLP is a consultant who provides assessment of vocal quality and vocal fold functioning. It is appropriate, however, to describe your structural findings as "suggestive of" or "consistent with" a particular disorder or pathology. (See a sample report on pages 47-48.)

The following is an example of reported finding of visual assessment:

> **Structural**: "The vocal folds present with areas of bilateral thickening at the one-third junction from the anterior commissure on the medial/vibratory margins. This finding is consistent with vocal fold nodules."

> **Functional**: "As a result, medial glottal closure is incomplete with reduced amplitude of vibration bilaterally. Mucosal wave is also mildly reduced."

## RECOMMENDATIONS

Offer recommendations based upon the results of the evaluation process. If you perform the voice evaluation independent of the ENT, appropriate recommendations may include "re-evaluation by ENT" or "review of examination with ENT for medical management."

If the evaluation is performed collaboratively, it is appropriate for you to report the recommendation made by the physician in addition to the therapeutic recommendations:

> "Surgical excision of L vocal fold polyp as recommended by Dr. X."

> "Post-operative voice rest and voice therapy has been discussed with this patient and therapy will be scheduled to start 10 days post-operative."

If voice therapy is recommended, include a diagnosis (use ICD-9 codes listed on page 49), specific number of sessions, and duration for approval/authorization by insurance:

> "Voice therapy is recommended, targeting remediation of vocal fold nodules 1x/week for 12 weeks."

# Protocol for Voice Evaluation

**Purpose**: The purpose of this policy is to describe the procedures used for objective data assessment of voice disordered clients.

**Scope**: The policy applies to all speech-language pathologists involved with the evaluation of voice disorders.

**Procedure**

1. Consult received from physician
2. Case history/speech pathology intake form to be reviewed with the patient
3. Completion of the *Voice Handicap Index* (VHI) by the patient
4. Objective measures will be obtained using the Computerized Speech Lab (CSL), maintaining a sampling rate of 50,000 and a microphone-to-mouth distance less than 10cm (optimal 3-4cm) at a 45-90 degree angle from the mouth for sustained productions to reduce airflow noise/breath contamination (as recommended by the Summary Statement Workshop on Acoustic Voice Analysis, NCVS 1994).

   ### Sustained Phonation
   /a/ = (3-4 second sample) at modal pitch and comfortable loudness
   - Analyze via MDVP (Multi-Dimensional Voice Program) to include all parameters and radial graph.
   - Report fundamental frequency, jitter %, shimmer (in dB), and H/N ratio. Use Baken and Orlikoff norms (1992).
   - Assess jitter on high /i/ and low /u/ vowel productions to assess source-vocal tract interactions. (Jitter reliability is high for type 1 signals only. Use all parameters [visual graph/MDVP] for type 2 & 3 signals.)

   ### Speech Samples
   a) Counting 1-10
   b) All-voiced sentence: "Where are you going?"
   c) Voice onset/offset: "The blue spot is on the key."

   - Analyze via RTP (Real Time Pitch) protocol for habitual pitch.
   - Report fundamental frequency and amplitude.
   - Use tasks b) and c) to assess adductory control.

   ### Pitch Range
   Instruct the patient to move from a comfortable pitch to the lowest and then to the highest.
   - Analyze via RTP protocol for pitch range.

   ### Maximum Phonation Time (MPT): average of two trials on sustained /a/

   ### S/Z Ratio
   sustained /s/ maximum duration
   sustained /z/ maximum duration

   ### Reading: Rainbow Passage
   assessment of breath support patterns during running speech and WPM (if appropriate)

5. Write report and attach all pertinent acoustic measures. Include diagnostic impressions (including ICD-9) and recommendations.

Proposed by Sandra Kasper Schwartz (Presbyterian Voice Center, University of Pennsylvania Health System June 2003)

# Case History Form

Patient _____

Parent/Guardian _____

Date of Birth _____  Age _____

Occupation _____

Name/Phone of physician who referred you _____

Please explain the problem for which you are being seen today.

_____

_____

_____

How long have you been experiencing this/these condition(s)? _____

Do you smoke? _____  If *yes*, how much? _____

Do you drink alcohol? _____  If *yes*, how much per week? _____

How much caffeine do you drink per day? _____

How much water do you drink per day? _____

List any medication(s) you are currently taking.

_____

_____

List any major surgeries and the approximate dates.

_____

_____

Have you ever been treated by an ENT (Ear, Nose & Throat) physician in the past? _____

If *yes*, for what condition(s)? _____

Have you ever been treated by a speech-language pathologist? _____

If *yes*, explain. _____

Are you a singer? _____

Have you received formal voice training in the past? _____

*continued on next page*

Do you currently experience or have history of any of the following?  (Please circle any that apply.)

high blood pressure
low blood pressure
heart attack
stroke
shortness of breath
asthma
frequent bronchitis
upper respiratory conditions
  (Explain _____ )
allergies
heartburn/gastroesophageal reflux
stomach ulcers
hiatal hernia
gastrointestinal conditions
  (Explain _____ )
cancer
  (Explain _____ )
TMJ
hearing loss

dry mouth
dry throat
frequent throat clearing
chronic cough
feeling of a "lump" in throat
difficulty swallowing
frequent laryngitis
frequent sore throats
voice change
throat tightness
fatigue after speaking
difficulty getting volume
loss of voice in morning
loss of voice at night

Other medical conditions not listed above

_____

_____

_____

Other changes related to your throat/voice

_____

_____

_____

_____        _____
Signature of Patient/Parent or Guardian              Date

# Effects of Medication on Voice/Speech

Clinicians within a medical setting should be familiar with the use of a PDR (Physician's Desk Reference) to check for side effects that may affect the voice or cause cough.

**Groups of medications that have documented negative effects on voice/speech**

- androgens
- anabolic steroids
- central nervous system stimulants
- sedatives
- narcotics
- tricyclic antidepressants
- inhaled steroids
- antihistamines
- (some) cardiovascular medications/ACE inhibitors
- anti-anxiety agents

**Groups that may have favorable effects on voice/speech**

- hydrating agents
- steroids
- acid inhibitors/Proton Pump Inhibitors (PPI)

Adapted from the National Center for Voice and Speech website on the "200 most frequently prescribed medication in the U.S." (11/99) *http://www.ncvs.org/ncvs/info/vocol/rx.html*

It is important to note medications when performing chart review and/or the intake interview with a patient/caregiver. Keep in mind:

- dosage and duration of use (Is the patient taking the medication as directed?)
- onset of speech/voice/cognitive change relative to start or cessation of medication
- drug interactions
- patient's age
- overall health/co-morbidity of other conditions that may cause or exacerbate symptoms

Speak with the physician regarding a possible change in dose or to different medication if you feel that symptoms might be drug induced. Consider changing the time medication is given to maximize desirable effects, such as reducing tremor (e.g., Sinemet) or reducing anxiety levels (e.g., Ativan) during periods of increased voice use.

# Consensus Auditory-Perceptual Evaluation of Voice (CAPE-V)

Name: _____   Date: _____

The following parameters of voice quality will be rated upon completion of the following tasks:

1.  Sustained vowels (/a/ and /i/) for 3-5 seconds duration each.

2.  Sentence production:

       a.  The blue spot is on the key again.    d.  We eat eggs every Easter.
       b.  How hard did he hit him?           e.  My mama makes lemon muffins.
       c.  We were away a year ago.          f.  Peter will keep at the peak.

3.  Spontaneous speech in response to "Tell me about your voice problem." or "Tell me how your voice is functioning."

```
Legend:   C = Consistent          I = Intermittent
          MI = Mildly Deviant
          MO = Moderately Deviant
          SE = Severely Deviant
```

SCORE

**Overall Severity** _____   C   I   _____/100
                MI        MO        SE

**Roughness** _____   C   I   _____/100
                MI        MO        SE

**Breathiness** _____   C   I   _____/100
                MI        MO        SE

**Strain** _____   C   I   _____/100
                MI        MO        SE

**Pitch** (Indicate the nature of the abnormality): _____
_____   C   I   _____/100
                MI        MO        SE

**Loudness** (Indicate the nature of the abnormality): _____
_____   C   I   _____/100
                MI        MO        SE

_____ _____   C   I   _____/100
                MI        MO        SE

_____ _____   C   I   _____/100
                MI        MO        SE

Comments about resonance:       normal       other  (Provide description):

_____

Additional features (e.g., diplophonia, fry, falsetto, asthenia, aphonia, pitch instability, tremor, wet/gurgly, or other relevant terms):

                                             Clinician: _____

# Voice Handicap Index (VHI)

Instructions: These are statements that many people have used to describe their voices and the effects of their voices on their lives. Circle the response that indicates how frequently you have the same experience.

**Never – 0    Almost Never – 1    Sometimes – 2    Almost Always – 3    Always – 4**

| | | Never | Almost Never | Sometimes | Almost Always | Always |
|---|---|---|---|---|---|---|
| F1. | My voice makes it difficult for people to hear me. | 0 | 1 | 2 | 3 | 4 |
| P2. | I run out of air when I talk. | 0 | 1 | 2 | 3 | 4 |
| F3. | People have difficulty understanding me in a noisy room. | 0 | 1 | 2 | 3 | 4 |
| P4. | The sound of my voice varies throughout the day. | 0 | 1 | 2 | 3 | 4 |
| F5. | My family has difficulty hearing me when I call them throughout the house. | 0 | 1 | 2 | 3 | 4 |
| F6. | I use the phone less often than I would like. | 0 | 1 | 2 | 3 | 4 |
| E7. | I'm tense when talking with others because of my voice. | 0 | 1 | 2 | 3 | 4 |
| F8. | I tend to avoid groups of people because of my voice. | 0 | 1 | 2 | 3 | 4 |
| E9. | People seem irritated with my voice. | 0 | 1 | 2 | 3 | 4 |
| P10. | People ask, "What's wrong with your voice?" | 0 | 1 | 2 | 3 | 4 |
| F11. | I speak with friends, neighbors, or relatives less often because of my voice. | 0 | 1 | 2 | 3 | 4 |
| F12. | People ask me to repeat myself when speaking face-to-face. | 0 | 1 | 2 | 3 | 4 |
| P13. | My voice sounds creaky and dry. | 0 | 1 | 2 | 3 | 4 |
| P14. | I feel as though I have to strain to produce voice. | 0 | 1 | 2 | 3 | 4 |
| E15. | I feel other people don't understand my voice problem. | 0 | 1 | 2 | 3 | 4 |
| F16. | My voice difficulties restrict my personal and social life. | 0 | 1 | 2 | 3 | 4 |
| P17. | The clarity of my voice is unpredictable. | 0 | 1 | 2 | 3 | 4 |
| P18. | I try to change my voice to sound different. | 0 | 1 | 2 | 3 | 4 |
| F19. | I feel left out of conversations because of my voice. | 0 | 1 | 2 | 3 | 4 |
| P20. | I use a great deal of effort to speak. | 0 | 1 | 2 | 3 | 4 |
| P21. | My voice is worse in the evening. | 0 | 1 | 2 | 3 | 4 |
| F22. | My voice problem causes me to lose income. | 0 | 1 | 2 | 3 | 4 |
| E23. | My voice problem upsets me. | 0 | 1 | 2 | 3 | 4 |
| E24. | I am less outgoing because of my voice problem. | 0 | 1 | 2 | 3 | 4 |
| E25. | My voice makes me feel handicapped. | 0 | 1 | 2 | 3 | 4 |
| P26. | My voice "gives out" on me in the middle of speaking. | 0 | 1 | 2 | 3 | 4 |
| E27. | I feel annoyed when people ask me to repeat. | 0 | 1 | 2 | 3 | 4 |
| E28. | I feel embarrassed when people ask me to repeat. | 0 | 1 | 2 | 3 | 4 |
| E29. | My voice makes me feel incompetent. | 0 | 1 | 2 | 3 | 4 |
| E30. | I'm ashamed of my voice problem. | 0 | 1 | 2 | 3 | 4 |

Note: The letter preceding each item corresponds to the subscale (E=emotional subscale, F=functional subscale, P=physical subscale)

*The Voice Handicap Index* (VHI): Development and Validation, Barbara H. Jacobson, Alex Johnson, Cynthia Grywalski, Alice Silbergleit, Gary Jacobson, Michael S. Benninger, *American Journal of Speech-Language Pathology*, Vol 6(3), 66-70, 1997. Reprinted with permission.

When the sunlight strikes raindrops in the air, they act like a prism and form a rainbow. The rainbow is a division of white light into many beautiful colors. These take the shape of a long round arch, with its path high above, and its two ends apparently beyond the horizon. There is, according to legend, a boiling pot of gold at one end. People look, but no one ever finds it. When a man looks for something beyond his reach, his friends say he is looking for the pot of gold at the end of the rainbow.

Reprinted by permission from Grant Fairbanks, *Voice and Articulation Drillbook* (2nd ed.). Published by Allyn and Bacon, 75 Arlington St., Boston, MA 02116. Copyright © 1960 by Pearson Education. Further reproduction prohibited without written permission from the publisher.

# Consent to Perform Videostroboscopy

Client Name: _____

I hereby consent to and authorize the performance of videostroboscopy for assessment of vocal fold structure and functioning to be performed at Duquesne University Speech-Language-Hearing Clinic.

*Initial*: _____

I consent to the administration of topical anesthetic, if required. I have no known allergies and/or medical conditions that prohibit the use of topical anesthetics.

*Initial*: _____

The nature and purpose of the procedures and the potential risks involved have been explained to me. Potential risks include allergic reaction to topical anesthetic, bleeding (transnasal endoscopy only), and/or temporary discomfort. No guarantee or assurance has been given by anyone as to the results that may be obtained.

*Initial*: _____

I understand that all information pertaining to services at Duquesne University Speech-Language-Hearing Clinic is kept confidential and will be made available to other professional personnel only after I have signed an Authorization to Send/Release Information form.

*Initial*: _____

Duquesne University Speech-Language-Hearing Clinic is part of the professional degree program in the Rangos School of Health Sciences at Duquesne University. I understand that student clinicians participate in and/or observe services under the supervision of the certified and licensed professional staff of the Department of Speech-Language Pathology. Further, I understand that audio and/or videotapes of sessions and other case information may be used in professional teaching.

*Initial*: _____

_____     _____
*Signature of Client/Parent or Guardian*                                *Date Signed*

Reprinted with permission of Duquesne University Speech-Language-Hearing Clinic

# Protocol for Videostroboscopy

**Purpose**: The purpose of this policy is to describe the procedures used for videostroboscopic assessment of vocal fold structure and functioning.

**Scope**: The policy applies to all speech-language pathologists involved with the performance of videostroboscopy.

**Procedure**
- All examinations will be performed with a disinfected endoscope.
- Disinfectant will be solution approved by the FDA for use in high-level disinfection (HLD).
- HLD procedures will follow recommended guidelines by OSHA and storage/disposal will follow manufacturer's guidelines.

1. Explain the procedure to the patient and/or caretaker and inquire about known allergies to topical anesthetic.
2. Position the patient for examination.
3. Place the laryngeal microphone or EGG sensors on the patient to trigger the stroboscopic light pulse.
4. Utilize Universal Precautions (e.g., alcohol prep to sensors, gloves).
5. Procedure must be completed by an ENT physician or licensed and certified speech-language pathologist trained in the procedure.
6. Videostroboscopy will be performed utilizing a rigid 70 degree and/or a flexible fiberoptic endoscope. Anesthetic will be administered only as needed for oral endoscopy and will always be administered for transnasal endoscopy.
7. During evaluation of vocal function, the patient will be asked to perform the following vocal tasks:
   > Phonate /i/
   > Increase and decrease pitch
   > Increase and decrease volume
   > Produce staccato /i/  ("ee ee ee")

   During flexible examination:
   > Hold breath at the laryngeal level (for count of 7)
   > Count from 1-10

8. Vocal fold functional parameters will be assessed using the Hirano and Bless (1993) model to report the following parameters:  symmetry, periodicity, glottic closure, amplitude, mucosal wave, vibration, FVF structure, and movement.

*Note:  In order to judge vibratory parameters, the fundamental frequency must be appropriately measured.

**Report**

Reports will include a laryngeal image which is most representative of the findings as well as all assessed parameters noted above.  Impressions will include both a structural description and functional diagnosis. Structural diagnoses will be reviewed by/with ENT physician.  Recommendations for voice therapy will include frequency and number of requested sessions.

Proposed by Sandra Kasper Schwartz (Presbyterian Voice Center, University of Pennsylvania Health System June 2003)

# Voice Evaluation Report

Patient X
DOB:
Medical record #:
Referring physician:
Date of Evaluation:

## History/Status

Ms. X is a 41-year-old female with a diagnosis of vocal fold nodules (per report from Dr. ENT). Past medical history is significant for diabetes (IDDM). Reported medication includes insulin injections. Patient reports voice has been hoarse for 1+ years and is worse in the a.m. Patient does not report dysphagia or odynophagia. Patient is a non-smoker and reports no alcohol intake. Patient reports symptoms associated with GERD (heartburn, belching) for which she takes antacids.

Patient is employed as a 4th grade teacher and therefore engages in excessive voice use daily.

## Evaluation

Vocal quality is mild-moderately harsh. Mild strain is also present upon production of sustained vocalization.

Voice parameters were quantified via computerized speech lab (CSL) (see MDVP radial graph on the next page):

- Sustained phonation of /a/ = 206.0 Hz; jitter = 4.1%; shimmer = .96dB; N/H = .28
- Pitch range = 199Hz low/315 Hz high
- Automatic speech (counting) = 188.8 Hz; 62.0dB
- All-voiced sentence production = 203.9 Hz / 61.4dB
- Voice/voiceless onsets = 187.8 Hz/58.9dB
- MPT = 10 sec.     s/z = 10/8 secs. = 1.25

Measurements reveal increased perturbation upon sustained phonation. Pitch range is mildly reduced. MPT is reduced suggestive of poor medial glottal closure. These findings are consistent with this patient's present diagnosis of vocal fold nodules.

## Videostroboscopy

A videostroboscopic examination was performed utilizing both a rigid and flexible endoscope. Assessment was performed both during sustained phonation /i/ and running speech.

The vocal folds present with areas of increased mass bilaterally at the $\frac{1}{3}$ junction from the anterior commissure. These areas make persistent vibratory contact during phonation and result in an anterior and posterior glottal gap. Vibration is periodic with mildly reduced amplitude of vibration and a mild-moderate reduction in mucosal wave propagation bilaterally. These areas of increased mass are consistent with a diagnosis of vocal fold nodules.

Moderate false vocal fold (FVF) tension is present upon phonation in an effort to obtain medial closure of the vocal folds. Arytenoid adduction and abduction are within functional limits (WFL). Mild interarytenoid thickening/hypertrophy is present and suggestive of gastro-esophageal reflux (GER) or laryngo-pharyngeal reflux (LPR).

**Impressions**

1. Hyperfunctional dysphonia with vocal fold nodules per ENT report.
2. Findings suggestive of GER/LPR irritation to the larynx.
3. Prognosis for improvement is positive with voice therapy.

**Recommendations**

1. Voice therapy (92507) 1x/week for 8 weeks for remediation of vocal fold nodules (478.5). See enclosed plan of treatment.
2. Pharmacological management of reflux (GER) symptoms such as use of a proton pump inhibitor (PPI) will be discussed with the referring physician. Reviewed dietary recommendations for control of reflux with the patient at the time of evaluation.
3. Consider use of classroom amplification.
4. Follow up with ENT post therapy as indicated.

_____

*Speech-Language Pathologist*

The Multi-Dimensional Voice Program (MDVP) is a software program available for the CSL (KAY Elemetrics) which acquires, analyzes, and displays a number of voice parameters analyzed during sustained phonation. This graph provides a visual representation with the patient's vocalization plotted against a circle representing the normative threshold values. (Refer to MDVP literature for parameter names and defined measures.)

This graphic display is useful to provide the patient with visual feedback regarding the degree of abnormality of the voice with respect to normative values, as well as to document change during the treatment process.

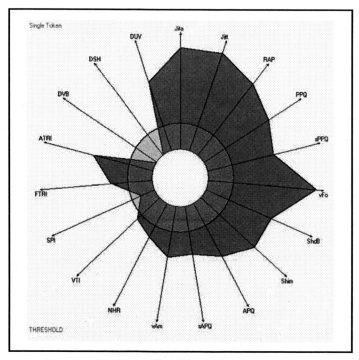

Courtesy of Kay Elemetrics Corp.

**The Source for Voice Disorders**
**Adolescent & Adult**
Copyright © 2004 LinguiSystems, Inc.

# ICD-9 Codes

The following ICD-9 codes are commonly used for voice disorders/pathologies:

| | |
|---|---|
| Aphonia | 784.41 |
| Cough | 786.2 |
| Dysphonia | 478.79 |
|     Functional | 300.11 |
|     Hysterical | 300.11 |
|     Psychogenic | 306.1 |
|     Spastic | 478.79 |
| Hoarseness | 784.49 |
| Laryngeal edema | 478.6 |
| Laryngeal spasms | 478.75 |
| Laryngitis (chronic) | 476.0 |
| Laryngitis (acute) | 464.0 |
| GER | 530.11 |
| Vocal fold | |
|     polyps | 478.4 |
|     other diseases (e.g., nodules, granuloma) | 478.5 |
| Vocal fold paralysis | |
|     unilateral | 478.31 |
|     bilateral | 478.34 |
| History of laryngeal cancer | V10.21 |

The term *voice disorders* encompasses a wide variety of medical, functional, and sometimes psychogenic diagnoses. Vocal disorders and pathologies may coexist and one may place the patient at risk for another. The speech-language pathologist should have a working knowledge of these sub-components that may precipitate or be the result of a vocal disorder or pathology. It is important to understand the condition for which the patient has been referred, possible underlying etiologies, and effects on structure and function of the vocal mechanism. This chapter provides reference material to help integrate medical and functional diagnoses, develop appropriate treatment, and identify the need for multi-disciplinary referrals.

A **disorder** is defined as "a disturbance of structure, function, or both."

A **pathology** is defined as "structural and functional changes that result from a disease process."

The terms *vocal pathology* and *voice disorder* are often used interchangeably because the structure and function of the vocal folds are directly related. It is the disturbance of structure and/or function that results in a "pathologic" voice.

The information in this chapter will help you classify voice disorders. The following categories have become widely accepted in the literature relating to voice nomenclature (Rosen & Murry 2000) and have been used in this chapter to organize disorders and pathologies:

- functional
- neurological
- organic

The chart on the next page categorizes voice diagnoses by their visual presentation and etiology. As noted later in this chapter, although a lesion's etiology may be functional, the resulting changes in vocal fold tissue place it as an organic pathology (e.g., nodules).

# Classification of Voice Disorders and Pathologies

| Functional | Neurological | Organic |
|---|---|---|
| functional aphonia | vocal fold paralysis | vocal fold nodule |
| paradoxical vocal fold movement (PVFM) | spasmodic dysphonia | polyp |
| muscle tension dysphonia (MTD) | | cyst |
| ventricular phonation | | granuloma |
| traumatic laryngitis | | contact ulcer |
| puberphonia | | infectious laryngitis |
| | | reflux laryngitis |
| | | presbylarynx |
| | | sulcus vocalis |
| | | Reinke's edema/polypoid degeneration |
| | | leukoplakia/erythroplakia |
| | | hyperkeratosis |
| | | papilloma |
| | | webbing |
| | | cancer |

Note: There are many neurological conditions that have significant effects on vocal quality but are not listed as primary neurological voice disorders. These conditions are listed as secondary disorders because the origin of the disturbance is not focal or primary to the larynx. These conditions include the following:

- Parkinson's disease (PD)
- amyotrophic lateral sclerosis (ALS)
- multiple sclerosis (MS)
- Huntington's disease (HD or Huntington's chorea)
- myasthenia gravis (MG)
- essential tremor
- pseudobulbar palsy
- bulbar palsy

This chapter covers specific disorders and pathologies along with information regarding possible etiologies, the resulting vocal quality/characteristics, and treatment/therapy suggestions. The suggested therapy tasks are provided as a starting point. This information is not meant to be a recipe or protocol for treatment of all patients falling into these diagnostic categories. Chapter 4, pages 85-139, provides a detailed description of therapy approaches and tasks most often used during voice therapy.

This chapter does not include acoustic parameters as you should relate gathered objective data to normative values rather than to a specific pathological "voice profile." There are many disorders that may have the same or similar acoustic and aerodynamic measures. See Chapter 2 for assessment/evaluation protocols. Keep in mind that you will need to add this data to your knowledge of presentations and etiologies presented below to aid in the diagnostic process.

## FUNCTIONAL VOICE DISORDERS

- functional aphonia
- paradoxical vocal fold movement (PVFM)
- muscle tension dysphonia (MTD)
- ventricular phonation
- traumatic laryngitis
- puberphonia

A functional voice disorder implies "normal" anatomy/structure with disordered or inappropriate use of the mechanism for voice production. These disorders can be hyperfunctional or hypofunctional in nature.

## Functional Aphonia (often called "conversional" or "psychogenic" aphonia)

### Presentation
The structure and function of the vocal folds is within normal limits (WNL), but the person is aphonic (unable to produce a voice).

### Etiology
There is no organic or physiologic cause for the patient's aphonia. It is often psychological or "stress-induced," with the possibility of positive reinforcement or gain associated with voice loss (e.g., unable to work, unable to lecture).

### Vocal characteristics
The patient presents with total aphonia or "whispered" phonation. However, vegetative vocal tasks (e.g., throat-clearing, coughing) are normal.

### Treatment
Most often treatment is solely voice therapy, which is highly effective in returning functional phonation. In some cases, psychological counseling and/or pharmacological treatments may be incorporated if there is an underlying functional etiology or onset event that is suspected to perpetuate or reinforce the voice loss.

### Therapy tasks
Very often voicing can be elicited in the first session through the use of vegetative tasks. For example, ask the patient to clear his throat and/or cough to elicit vocal "noise." Then use vegetative "uh-huh" or "mmm-hmm" in response to "yes" questions.

**Example**:

Clinician: "Is your name _____?"
Patient: "Uh-huh."
Clinician: "Is today _____?"
Patient: "Uh-huh."

Then carry the patient through a series of vocal tasks from the list below.

- humming—Have the patient produce a steady hum at a comfortable pitch and loudness.
- pitch glides using a hum—Have the patient produce a low-pitched and then high-pitched hum. Use pitch scales to go from low to higher pitches.
- resonance—/m/ words and sentences (pages 126-129)
- continuous voiced words (page 114)
- voicing—/v/ and /z/ phrases and sentences (page 115)

Once the patient is able to produce a stable voice on words and phrases using voiced consonants to elicit vibration (as described above), focus on longer utterances such as:

- paragraph reading
- conversation (structured and unstructured)
- dialogues to establish vocal variability
- poetry reading to practice prosodic variation

### Carryover tasks

At the completion of therapy, observe the patient in tasks such as telephone use, out-of-clinic environments, and with unfamiliar listeners in order to insure maintenance of the voice.

## Paradoxical Vocal Fold Movement (PVFM)
(often called *functional asthma* or *glottic dysfunction*)

### Presentation
Laryngeal structures and appearance are within normal limits (WNL); however, there is abnormal/paradoxical motion of the vocal folds, specifically adduction of vocal folds on inhalation.

### Etiology
This disorder is often misdiagnosed as asthma or an allergy symptom (e.g., cough, "wheeze"). The cause is still largely unknown, although it is believed to be triggered by anxiety or stress.

### Vocal characteristics
Resulting vocal symptoms include intermittent stridor, a strained vocal quality, and a non-productive cough.

### Treatment
Voice therapy has been advocated in the literature (Mathers-Schmidt 2001, Sandage & Zelazny 2004, Koufman & Block 2008) to "retrain" normal adductory and abductory movements during phonation and breathing.

Note: Obtain an ENT or pulmonary evaluation to insure "normal," non-obstructed upper airway before initiating therapy.

**Therapy tasks**

Focus on re-establishment of normal tidal breathing and airflow with accompanied phonation. The following tasks are suggested to promote laryngeal relaxation, airflow release, and coordinated breath support:

- diaphragmatic breathing (page 104)
- inhalation/exhalation practice (page 105)
- nasal inspiration—deep slow inhalation through the nose
- negative practice
    - holding breath at laryngeal level/Valsalva and release—Ask the patient to take a breath and "stop the air" on the way out by "bearing down."
    - ingressive phonation (phonating on inhalation)—Ask the patient to make a vocal noise with air coming in during inhalation.
- rapid adduction exercises (page 103a)
- airflow practice
    - /h/ words, phrases, and sentences (pages 109-111)
    - /f/ and /s/ phrases and sentences (pages 112-113)
- voiceless consonant words (page 118)
- coordination of airflow (page 107)

Once vocal strain is reduced and stridor is eliminated (both subjectively and through patient report), use increasingly demanding vocal tasks, such as the following:

- sentence of increasing length (page 108)
- paragraph reading for phrasing practice
- unstructured reading
- conversation

**Carryover tasks**

Throughout the therapy process, encourage the patient to practice target breathing techniques during activity (e.g., walking, exercising) to carry over this breathing pattern during increasing respiration.

# Muscle Tension Dysphonia (MTD)

MTD is commonly used in voice diagnosis to describe excessive muscle tension associated with phonation. The following classification is used as an additional descriptor of the type and degree of tension seen upon videostroboscopic examination:

**Classifications of MTD** (Koufman & Blalock 1991)

MTD type 1: posterior commissure is open (posterior gap) with reduced mucosal wave

MTD type 2: false vocal fold (FVF) approximation/adduction

MTD type 3: partial anterior-posterior (AP) constriction of the supraglottis

MTD type 4: complete supraglottic "squeeze" of the larynx (FVF and AP tension)

## Presentation
During phonation, there is hyperfunctional adduction/squeezing of the false vocal folds (FVF) and/or supraglottis.

## Etiology
Laryngeal structures may be normal or there may be an underlying pathology inhibiting vibration of the true vocal folds (TVFs) and/or creating "stiffness." (Presbylarynx or a medial glottal gap may also promote use of the FVFs to aid in medial closure.)

## Vocal characteristics
The voice most often presents with a reduced/low pitch and a strained vocal quality (may vary from mildly to severely strained).

## Treatment
Voice therapy is targeted at laryngeal relaxation during phonation.
Note: MTD type 4 may also be called *ventricular phonation* (page 56) and therefore benefits from similar therapy techniques.

## Therapy tasks
Focus on laryngeal relaxation through the use of easy phonatory tasks and the establishment of increased oral and nasal resonance (i.e., focus the voice away from the larynx) as highlighted in the following therapy tasks:

- cervical exercises (pages 97-100)
- diaphragmatic breathing (page 104)
- laryngeal massage techniques (page 91)—Use with MTD types 3 and 4.
- tactile vibration (page 125)
- humming—Have the patient produce a steady hum at a comfortable pitch and loudness.
- humming with pitch glides—Have the patient produce a low-pitched and then high-pitched hum. Use pitch scales to go from low to higher pitches.
- resonance focus (nasal) (page 126)
- /m/ words, phrases, and sentences (pages 126-131)
- resonance focus (oral) (page 130)
- /h/ words, phrases, and sentences (pages 109-111)
- /f/ and /s/ sentences (pages 112-113)
- easy onset of vowels (pages 119-120)
- tense vowels in words and phrases (page 131)

## Carryover tasks
Use longer passages and paragraphs to maintain relaxed voicing during tasks like the following:

- vowel intense paragraph (page 121)
- functional reading (e.g., magazine, newspaper) to promote use of relaxed voice in less structured tasks

## Ventricular Phonation (false vocal fold [FVF] adduction)

### Presentation
Complete adduction or closure of the FVFs/ventricular folds during phonation.

### Etiology
Laryngeal structures may be normal or there may be an underlying pathology or organic cause (same as MTD, pages 54-55).

### Vocal characteristics
The voice is often described as having a "pressed" or strained quality, often with a reduction of pitch.

### Treatment
Voice therapy is targeted at the release of supraglottic/FVF adduction and maintenance of a relaxed laryngeal posture.

Note: Obtain an ENT evaluation to rule out any underlying vocal fold pathology prior to initiating therapy.

### Therapy tasks
Promote laryngeal relaxation during vibratory voicing tasks ("easy voicing") and establish increased oral and nasal resonance. The following tasks are recommended:

- cervical exercises (pages 97-100)
- palatal stretching (page 95)
- laryngeal massage techniques (page 91)
- tactile vibration (page 125)
- humming—Have the patient produce a steady hum at a comfortable pitch and loudness.
- humming with pitch glides—Have the patient produce a low-pitched and then high-pitched hum. Use pitch scales to go from low to higher pitches.
- resonance focus (pages 125-126)
- /m/ words, phrases, and sentences (pages 127-129)
- voiced vs. voiceless minimal pairs (pages 116-117)
- airflow practice
    - /h/ words, phrases, and sentences (pages 109-111)
    - /f/ and /s/ sentences (pages 112-113)
- continuous voiced words (page 114)
- "easy" vibration with /z/ and /v/ phrases and sentences (page 115)

### Carryover tasks
Target paragraph reading (both structured and unstructured) and conversation using "easy phonatory" techniques in the exercises listed above. Use magazines, books, and other functional reading materials followed by discussion.

## Traumatic Laryngitis (voice loss caused by abuse or irritation)

### Presentation
The vocal folds present with swelling (edema) and often redness (erythema) or increased vascularity (appearance of tiny blood vessels), resulting in "stiffness" and reduced vibration.

### Etiology
Onset may include a traumatic functional event (e.g., screaming at a football game, singing loudly at a concert) or may be induced by an irritant (e.g., chemical exposure, smoke inhalation).

### Vocal characteristics
The voice may present with varying degrees of dysphonia to complete aphonia ("total laryngitis").

### Treatment
The patient should be instructed to engage in a period of strict voice rest (1-3 days or until the voice is restored to its baseline quality). Any exposure to irritants should be eliminated if possible (e.g., wear a mask to reduce exposure, remove chemicals) and the patient should be instructed to keep well hydrated by increasing water intake. Steroids can be prescribed by a physician to reduce acute inflammation.

### Recommendations for the patient
Do not to try to "talk through" or "above" the laryngitis. Avoid straining your voice to talk. (Often complete voice rest is advised for a brief period, such as two to three days.) Do not whisper. Whispering results in increased vocal tension and increased airflow pressure that may further injure the vocal folds. Drink plenty of water to lubricate the vocal folds.

### Therapy tasks
In most cases of traumatic laryngitis, voice rest alone is sufficient to reduce the swelling and return the voice to its baseline quality. After a period of voice rest, if the "laryngitis" persists, it is advisable to repeat visualization of the larynx.

In some cases, acute laryngitis from trauma can result in a hemorrhage (bleed) of a vocal fold. This condition is often seen in singers or performers who have had a "heavy" practice or performance schedule. Risk of vocal fold hemorrhage increases with the use of aspirin products and, therefore, aspirin should be avoided if possible. (See page 135 for recommendations for singers.)

## Puberphonia ("mutational falsetto")

### Presentation
Puberphonia is most often seen in males. The larynx and vocal folds present with normal structure. During phonation, excessive tension is produced through lengthening of the vocal folds as seen in higher pitches with poor vibratory contact/medial closure ("falsetto voice").

### Etiology

Puberphonia is often considered to be psychosocial in origin; however, growth, hormonal, and endocrine disorders must be ruled out. (It is recommended that the patient be examined by his primary physician for a complete physical exam and to assess endocrine levels, in addition to being seen by the ENT physician to insure normal laryngeal structure prior to the onset of voice therapy.)

### Vocal characteristics

The voice presents with an abnormally high-pitched vocal quality for the person's age and expected norms (e.g., a male voice that has not "changed" post-puberty). Pitch breaks and vocal instability/poor voice control is also a characteristic.

Note: During puberty, the fundamental frequency/pitch drops approximately two to three notes in women and one octave in men. (For adult norms, see Chapter 2, page 26.)

### Treatment

Voice therapy targets the establishment of a vocal tone/pitch that is WNL for age and sex. Sometimes psychological counseling is recommended if psychosocial issues are believed to be related to the vocal quality.

### Therapy tasks

Initiate therapy with the use of vegetative phonatory tasks to elicit a lower pitch (e.g., throat-clearing, vocalized sigh). Once elicited during non-speech tasks, reinforce the practice of a "new" deeper vocal tone during speaking tasks like those listed below:

- Vegetative tasks
    throat-clearing—Ask the patient to clear his throat.
    "uh-huh"—Ask the patient to say affirmative "uh-huh" to "yes" questions.
    sigh—Vocalize a deep sigh ("Take a deep breath and then sigh out loud.")
- Pitch glides using a hum—Have the patient produce a low-pitched and then high-pitched hum. Use pitch scales to go from low to higher pitches.
- Pitch manipulation tasks/comparative pitch drills—Have the patient say "ee" at a high pitch and then "ah" at a low pitch.
- Digital manipulation to lower the larynx (performed by the SLP or patient)—Place fingers on the superior horns of the thyroid cartilage and push gently inward and downward while phonating to elicit a lower laryngeal posture.
- Reading words and phrases at a "low pitch" vs. "high pitch"—Have the patient repeat the same word/phrase and cue him to use a "deep voice" vs. "squeaky voice" to contrast pitch and reinforce the ability to "change your voice." Then read the target words/phrases using only the "deep voice."

### Carryover tasks

Work toward maintenance of a lower pitch during words, sentences, paragraphs, and finally conversation. At the completion of therapy, make recordings of the patient's voice. Listening to his new voice will help the patient accept this "deeper" vocal quality.

Note: During therapy, maximum encouragement and reinforcement of the newly established vocal quality is often needed. The patient needs to understand the process of voice change and feel as if he has gained "control" over his voice.

## NEUROLOGICAL VOICE DISORDERS

- vocal fold paralysis
- spasmodic dysphonia

A neurological voice disorder results from an interruption in neuromuscular control, causing reduced, uncoordinated, or absent movement of laryngeal structures.

# Vocal Fold Paralysis

### Presentation
Vocal fold motion is impaired during adduction and abduction. The affected vocal fold(s)/arytenoid may be "fixed" in the medial, paramedian (partially abducted), or fully abducted position, and the paralysis may be unilateral or bilateral.

### Etiology
Possible insults resulting in vocal fold paralysis include damage to or compression of the recurrent laryngeal nerve (RLN) from a surgical procedure or a mass/tumor pressing along the course of the nerve. Other etiologies include viral infections that "attack" the nerve, or idiosyncratic onsets in which no precipitating event or injury occurred.

### Unilateral
This is the most common form of vocal fold paralysis, resulting from a disease or trauma to the RLN. The RLN is prone to surgical trauma because of the course in the neck and chest. (See page 16.) Unilateral impairment of the RLN affects innervation of the lateral cricoarytenoid on the affected side and results in an adductor paralysis with the vocal fold in paramedian position.

Diagnosis for patients presenting with a unilateral VF paralysis involves assessment via a CT scan of the neck and chest to rule out malignancy involving or compressing the RLN.

### Vocal characteristics
The voice presents with a harsh quality that is sometimes predominately breathy due to poor medial contact of the vocal folds during phonation. In some cases, a diplophonic quality is present, resulting from unequal tension on the folds.

### Treatment
Many idiopathic or traumatic occurrences of vocal fold paralysis demonstrate spontaneous recovery in the first 6-12 months. Interim treatment may involve voice therapy to improve medial compensation and breath support for voicing. (Patients may also benefit from a head rotation to the affected side to improve medial closure of the vocal folds for speech and swallowing.)

Temporary surgical intervention may be performed to allow for improved medial closure, including injections of autologous fat, collagen, synthetic material (Gelfoam), or processed human tissue (Cymetra). These substances add bulk to the lateral margins of the paralyzed vocal fold improving medialization for vocal fold contact. These materials are reabsorbed by the body with results lasting an average of three to six months and, therefore, their effects are considered temporary. A newer material approved by the FDA for vocal fold augmentation is Calcium hydroxylapatite (abbreviated CaHA) (trade name Radiesse). It is being used with longer lasting effects (approximately one to two years).

After the designated post-onset period without evidence of recovery, options for permanent surgical intervention include medialization thyroplasty. Thyroplasty involves a surgical excision into the thyroid cartilage to create a window in which a silicone wedge is placed to "push" the vocal fold into midline. This procedure may also be performed with a graft of cartilage taken from elsewhere in the body (e.g., nasal cartilage).

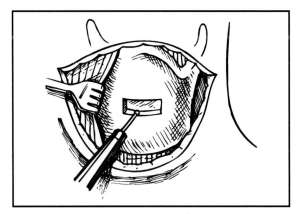

Figure 23.  Surgical creation of thyroid window

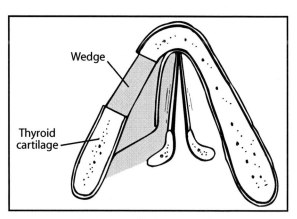

Figure 24.  Placement of silicone wedge

### Bilateral
In cases of bilateral vocal fold paralysis, the injury is usually the result of a brain stem infarct also resulting in weakness or paralysis of the velum, tongue, and pharyngeal constrictors.

### Vocal characteristics
In cases of bilateral *adductor* paralysis, the resulting voice is severely breathy or aphonic because the vocal folds are in an open position (abducted). In contrast, in bilateral *abductor* paralysis, the vocal folds are in the midline or closed (adducted) position, resulting in stridor and shortness of breath. This condition may be a medical emergency.

### Treatment
Breathing and swallowing are often severely impaired in cases of bilateral vocal fold paralysis resulting from a brain stem infarct. Treatment for bilateral *abductor* paralysis typically involves tracheostomy to insure a patent airway. A one-way speaking valve (e.g., Passy-Muir) may be placed if the patient is judged to be an adequate candidate from a respiratory standpoint. These patients often get adequate voicing because the vocal folds remain in an approximated position.

In cases of bilateral *adductor* paralysis, the physician may choose to perform a unilateral thyroplasty to allow one vocal fold to be midline. This procedure allows for some voicing and assists with airway protection for swallowing as long as the airway remains open for breathing.

### Therapy Tasks

These patients are typically managed medically for the voice as described above. As an SLP, you are most often involved to assist with speaking valve placement and/or to rehabilitate swallowing.

## Spasmodic Dysphonia (SD)

### Presentation

SD involves spasms of the arytenoids and true vocal folds, and may include the false vocal folds and pharyngeal constrictors. In severe cases, neck and shoulder movements as well as facial grimacing may be involved. Patients will often display emotional symptoms of anxiety or depression related to their voices.

Alternative diagnoses, which may have similar presentations to SD and should be considered during the process of differential diagnosis of SD, include essential vocal tremor, amyotrophic lateral sclerosis (ALS or Lou Gehrig's disease), muscle tension dysphonia (MTD), Parkinson's, and psychogenic dysphonia.

### Etiology

Currently the etiology is unknown. Previously, SD was considered to be of psychological origin, however current research using diagnostic procedures such as PET scans, EEG, and laryngeal EMG suggest a neurological origin (Dedo et al. 1978, Aminoff et al. 1978, Blitzer & Brin 1992).

### Vocal characteristics

Vocal quality is strained with voice breaks or phonatory arrests due to an interruption of airflow by the vocal folds. Changes in glottal airflow may result in excessive volume, intermittent breathiness, and audible inhalation. See below for vocal characteristics associated with specific types of SD.

### *Types of SD*

**Adductor SD** is the most common type of SD. It involves involuntary contraction of the adductors during phonation, resulting in the following vocal characteristics:
- strained-strangled voice
- abrupt onset and phonatory breaks, sudden interruption of voicing
- increase in tension and changes in loudness (most often observed during sustained vowel production)

**Abductor SD** involves involuntary contraction of the abductors that separate the vocal folds during phonation (posterior cricoarytenoid muscle, see pages 8-9) and the inability to sustain glottal closure, resulting in the following vocal characteristics:
- breathiness
- reduction of speaking pitch
- delay in voice onsets (most often observed as interruptions or delay in transition from voiceless to voiced phonemes)

Mixed SD presents with involuntary movements of both adductory and abductory muscles. This type of SD may result in any combination of the vocal characteristics discussed on page 61.

**Medical treatment**

The most common treatment of SD involves the use of Botox (Botulinum Toxin) injections.

Botox is produced by a bacterium that, in very large doses, can be toxic. However, when prepared/activated under controlled conditions and injected in small doses, it has proven to be medically beneficial in the treatment of many dystonias (e.g., blephorospasm, torticollis). Botox works by blocking acetylcholine that transmits messages across neuromuscular junctions. Simply stated, it is a nerve impulse blocker. When injected into a target muscle that is "overactive," it weakens the contraction of the muscle, thereby controlling the spasm.

Botox has been approved for medical use by the FDA (Dec. 2000).

Use for Adductor SD: injection into the TA (thyroarytenoid)
Use for Abductor SD: injection into the PCA (posterior cricoarytenoid)

Therapeutic effects (helpful to share with patients):
- Patients will become breathy within five days of the injection. Breathiness may last up to two weeks.
- There is a risk for aspiration for up to two weeks post injection.
- When breathy vocal quality resolves, the voice returns without spasms; however it may have reduced volume.
- Effects of Botox are temporary, lasting two to four months on the average. Repeat injections are often needed.

Sectioning of the recurrent laryngeal nerve (RLN section) has also been used in cases of adductor SD. Unilateral section of the RLN will produce a unilateral vocal fold paralysis in the paramedian (slightly abducted) position, thereby weakening the voice (Dedo 1976).

The most effective form of treatment is often a combination of Botox and voice therapy (Murry & Woodson 1995). A brief course of voice therapy is often effective at reducing hyperfunctional compensatory behaviors and optimizing the effects of the Botox injections.

**Therapy tasks**

Therapy for SD should incorporate the following goals:

- focus on placement of the voice to reduce laryngeal focus
- improve vocal onsets (reduction of glottal attack)
- improve parameters such as rate and loudness

Note: You may also need to deal with social-emotional communication issues in therapy related to the patient's "loss of control" of his voice. Sometimes emotional or psychological counseling is recommended to assist with the anxiety that is often associated with this disorder.

## ORGANIC VOICE PATHOLOGIES

- vocal fold nodule
- polyp
- cyst
- granuloma
- contact ulcer
- infectious laryngitis
- reflux laryngitis
- presbylarynx
- sulcus vocalis
- Reinke's edema/polypoid degeneration
- leukoplakia/erythroplakia
- hyperkeratosis
- papilloma
- webbing
- cancer

An organic vocal pathology results in anatomic or histological change to laryngeal tissue, resulting in vocal dysfunction. Most organic pathologies are treated medically and/or surgically followed by post-operative voice rest and voice therapy. See pages 136-139 for example treatment plans.

### Pathologies Treated Medically and/or Therapeutically

- vocal fold nodules
- infectious laryngitis
- reflux laryngitis
- presbylarynx

## Vocal Fold Nodules (historically called *singer's* or *screamer's nodes*)

### Presentation
Vocal fold nodules are benign, focal lesions of the superficial lamina propria (see Figure 18, page 19). They are bilateral and most often located at the $\frac{1}{3}$ to $\frac{1}{2}$ junction from the anterior commissure on the medial or vibratory margin of the vocal folds. Nodules are often compared to callouses of the vocal fold(s) caused by chronic irritation and, therefore, there is fibrosis of the epithelium (which may vary in density). Early onset nodules are relatively soft and become increasing fibrotic with ongoing irritation.

### Etiology
Nodules are hyperfunctional (caused by persistent abuse and/or misuse of the voice). Unilateral nodule or thickening may occur as the result of a lesion (cyst or polyp) on the contralateral (opposite) vocal fold, making persistent vibratory contact during phonation. This is called a *reactive nodule.*

**Effects on vocal function and voice production**
Due to the location of the nodules, poor medial glottal closure (usually an anterior and posterior gap/hourglass closure) may result in breathiness/ harshness. Hoarseness is a result of interruptions in vibration and mucosal wave, which may or may not be present, depending on the size of the nodules and degree of fibrosis. The most common patient complaints include hoarseness and vocal fatigue.

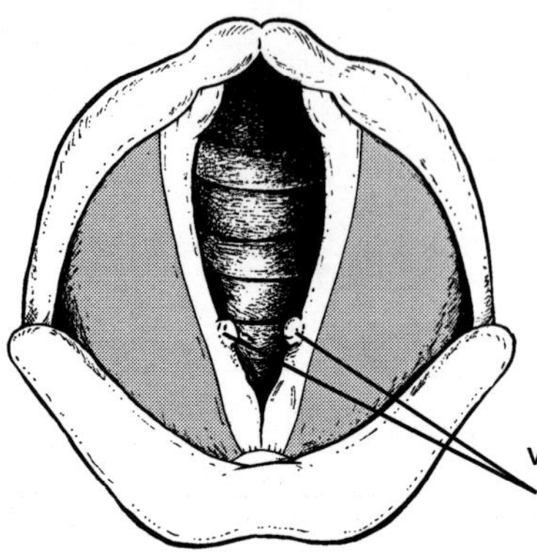

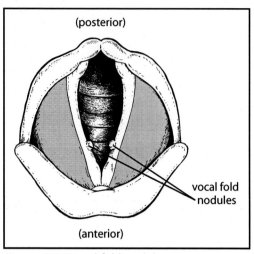

Figure 25. Vocal fold nodules

**Treatment**
Vocal nodules are the most common organic vocal pathology referred for voice therapy. Nodules are the only organic pathology listed in this text that is often successfully treated with voice therapy alone.

Treatment should be initiated with a program of vocal hygiene and increased hydration (page 88). Therapy should incorporate activities similar to those reviewed for other hyperfunctional disorders (e.g., MTD, ventricular phonation) with the focus to relieve vocal hyperfunction. The following are suggested therapy tasks:

- cervical exercises (pages 97-100)
- diaphragmatic breathing (page 104)
- airflow practice and tension monitoring (page 109)
- /h/ words, phrases, and sentences (pages 109-111)
- /f/ and /s/ sentences (pages 112-113)
- resonance focus (nasal) (pages 125-126)
- /m/ words, phrases, and sentences (pages 127-129)
- resonance focus (oral) (page 130)
- continuous voice words (page 114)
- voiced and voiceless transitions (pages 116-118)
- easy onset of vowels (pages 119-120)
- tense vowels in words and phrases (page 131)

**Carryover tasks**
Use longer passages and paragraphs to maintain relaxed voicing during tasks like the following:

- sentences of increasing length (page 108) to coordinate airflow and easy phonation
- vowel intense paragraph (page 121)
- functional reading (e.g., magazines, newspapers) to promote use of relaxed voice in less structured tasks

## Infectious Laryngitis

### Presentation
The vocal folds present with bilateral edema (swelling) and erythema (redness). Hypervascularity (increased appearance of tiny blood vessels) may also be present, resulting from "strain" in an effort to produce voice.

### Etiology
Loss of voice/laryngitis results from a bacterial infection of the upper respiratory tract (URI).

### Effects on vocal function and voice production
The degree of hoarseness will vary from mild dysphonia to complete aphonia based on the degree of inflammation. This increase in mass (swelling) results in stiffness and a reduced mucosal wave. Inflammation may be exacerbated by a possible cough associated with URI.

Repeated bouts of laryngitis (laryngeal inflammation) and cough may place the patient at risk for epithelial changes, such as vocal fold nodules.

### Treatment
Treatment is medical and may include prescribed antibiotics for treatment of the URI and in some cases steroids to reduce acute inflammation. A period of voice rest (2-5 days) may be recommended to reduce vocal strain and facilitate healing.

## Reflux Laryngitis

### Presentation
Bilateral edema (swelling), erythema (redness), and increased vascularity of the vocal folds may be present as in infectious laryngitis. However, edema of the posterior glottis and possible hypertrophy (proliferation of tissue) in the interarytenoid and/or post-cricoid space (also called *pachydermia laryngis*) is characteristic of inflammation resulting from esophageal acid exposure. Koufman (1991) also reports findings of a pseudosulcus (furrow or scar) at the vocal processes and obliteration of the ventricles (poor ability to visualize the ventricular space due to edema).

### Etiology
Reflux laryngitis results from gastro-esophageal acid that flows back up, reaching the level of the larynx. This is also termed *laryngo-pharyngeal reflux* (LPR) (see pages 73-76).

### Effects on vocal function and voice production
Hoarseness is present in varying degrees and is usually worse in the morning. Reported symptoms often include the presence of a dry, nonproductive cough (that is often greater when lying down) and chronic throat clearing. Other symptoms include a globus sensation (lump in throat) and dysphagia or odynophagia (pain upon swallowing), which is the result of posterior laryngeal swelling.

Repeated exposure to GER places the patient at risk for epithelial changes (e.g., granulomas, contact ulcers) and increases the risk for esophageal cancer.

**Treatment**

Medications are often prescribed to inhibit or reduce excess acid production. These include classifications of medication called *H2 blockers* or *proton-pump inhibitors (PPIs)*. Besides medication, dietary and lifestyle modifications should be recommended (see pages 75-76).

Reflux laryngitis is most often a chronic condition and, therefore, patients should be monitored to assess inflammation of the laryngeal structures, especially patients who experience persistent hoarseness.

A short course of therapy (one or two therapy sessions) is often recommended to provide and review acid reflux precautions and initiate dietary changes (see handout, page 76).

# Presbylarynx

**presbylarynx**:  physiological changes to the vocal fold(s), resulting in atrophy/bowing of the muscle

**presbyphonia**:  vocal quality resulting from and associated with the aging voice

**Presentation**

The vocal folds present with a bowed or atrophic (thin) appearance, often resulting in a medial glottal gap during phonation.

**Etiology**

Many changes take place in the cartilage, blood supply, connective tissue, and secretions of the aging laryngeal structures. These changes include ossification of the cartilage, arthritic changes of the joints, loss of elasticity, and increased fibrosis of the tissues, as well as atrophy of the muscles.

**Effects on vocal function and voice production**

The changes in laryngeal physiology noted above may affect the movement, control, and vibratory characteristics of the vocal folds, resulting in a weak or breathy quality to the voice. Sometimes patients complain of poor control or a generalized instability of their voices.

**Treatment**

In some cases of severe atrophy with poor medial closure/glottal incompetence, aspiration may be a risk. In those patients, or in patients whose change in vocal quality affects their abilities to communicate effectively or maintain quality of life, surgical procedures may be performed. Surgical injections similar to those used for vocal fold paralysis (page 59) including collagen, autologous fat, and synthetic materials (Gelfoam) are used to add bulk or mass to the vocal folds.

Voice therapy is the preferred treatment for most patients. Exercises should focus on improving breath support, medial glottal closure, pitch control, and vocal flexibility. Suggested therapy tasks are listed on the next page.

- adduction exercises (pages 101-102)
- rapid adduction exercises (page 103a)
- pitch glides using an /a/ or /i/ vowel—Have the patient produce low-pitched and high-pitched vowel sounds. Use pitch scales to go from low to higher pitches.
- diaphragmatic breathing (page 104)
- breath support and airflow coordination (pages 105-107)

**Pathologies Treated Surgically**

The pathologies most often treated surgically include, but are not limited to, the following:

- vocal fold polyps
- vocal fold cysts
- granulomas
- contact ulcers
- Reinke's edema
- laryngeal papilloma
- laryngeal web
- sulcus vocalis
- hyperkeratosis
- leukoplakia and erythroplakia
- cancer

The surgical procedure is called *microlaryngoscopy* or *phonosurgery*. The goal of phonosurgical techniques is to minimally disrupt the glottal margin and preserve mucosa to allow for full return of the vibratory properties and movement of the mucosal wave.

Patients should always be advised to engage in a period of vocal rest post-operatively to optimize the healing process. Although the duration of recommended vocal rest varies, an average of four to seven days is typically advised. Patients should also be instructed not to whisper during this time.

Post-operative voice rest and voice therapy are often incorporated into the treatment of these disorders and are used to reduce the presence of any identified behavioral or hyperfunctional behaviors that may contribute to the development and/or recurrence of the pathology.

## Vocal Fold Polyps and Cysts

Differential diagnosis of cysts vs. polyps is often a difficult one as the etiology and presentations are similar (see below and page 68). However, this distinction is not always a critical one as treatment is the same for both types of lesions. Both vocal fold cysts and polyps are most often removed surgically with post-operative voice therapy.

## Vocal Fold Polyps

### Presentation
Polyps are benign, focal lesions of the superficial lamina propria (sometimes slightly deeper), typically on the medial or vibratory margin of the vocal fold. They are most often unilateral (often with a reactive area of thickening contralaterally) and appear as soft, fluid-filled

(translucent) lesions. The point of attachment can be pedunculated (narrow point of attachment) or broad-based.

### Etiology
The development of a vocal fold polyp is hyperfunctional and may be a single abusive vocal event like coughing or screaming.

### Effects on vocal function and voice production
As a result of increased medial mass, poor glottal closure is achieved, resulting in breathiness or glottal air escape. A diplophonic quality is often present caused by differential mass and asymmetry of vibration bilaterally. Patients sometimes engage in throat-clearing due to a "tickle" in the throat from excessive vibration during phonation.

### Treatment (same for cysts and polyps)
Most often, surgical excision of the lesion is recommended. Pre-operative voice rest and vocal hygiene may be attempted in an effort to reduce the size of the lesion. Post operatively, voice rest is recommended for approximately 3-5 days, followed by a brief course of voice therapy. Therapy should target the identification and remediation of hyperfunctional or abusive vocal behaviors.

Voice therapy is essential when there is a contralateral reactive lesion/nodule. These unilateral "nodules" are often not excised during the surgery in an effort to reduce excision of the vocal folds. They are treated therapeutically the same as vocal fold nodules (page 63).

## Vocal Fold Cysts

### Presentation
Cysts are benign, focal lesions of the superficial lamina propria (submucosal or subepithelial) but may be deeper to the level of the vocalis (intracordal). They are most often unilateral (often with a reactive area of thickening contralaterally) and appear as soft, gelatinous lesions. The point of attachment is broad-based.

### Etiology
The development of vocal fold cysts result from vocal abuse or misuse that is chronic (less likely to be a single event).

### Effects on vocal function and voice production
Cysts are a slightly more dense lesion (gelatinous) and are reported to cause a greater reduction in mucosal wave than polyps. Cysts presenting deeper within the vocal fold structure (intracordal) more severely affect the vibration of the vocal fold. The resulting voice is hoarse and sometimes breathy. These patients are less likely to be diplophonic than patients with vocal fold polyps.

### Treatment (same for cysts and polyps)
Most often, surgical excision of the lesion is recommended. Pre-operative voice rest and vocal hygiene may be attempted in an effort to reduce the size of the lesion. Post operatively, voice rest is recommended for approximately 3-5 days, followed by a brief course of voice therapy.

Therapy should target the identification and remediation of hyperfunctional or abusive vocal behaviors.

Voice therapy is essential when there is a contralateral reactive lesion/nodule. These unilateral "nodules" are often not excised during the surgery in an effort to reduce excision of the vocal folds. They are treated therapeutically the same as vocal fold nodules (page 63).

# Granuloma

### Presentation
Granuloma appear most always posteriorly on the vocal processes. They appear consistent with hard granulation tissue that becomes epithelialized (irregular collection of tissue) into a formed mass. They usually present unilateral and can vary greatly in size.

### Etiology
The most common causes of granuloma include intubation, trauma or abuse, and/or gastroesophageal reflux (GER), resulting in irritation or damage to the mucosal perichondrium of the vocal process of the arytenoid cartilage.

### Effects on vocal function and voice production
Many granuloma do not affect vocal quality due to the location on the cartilaginous (non-vibratory) portion of the vocal fold. Some patients with larger granuloma present with hoarseness and/or breathiness, resulting from an inability to gain medial closure of the vocal folds. Chronic throat-clearing is often a vocal symptom.

### Treatment
Granuloma are often recurrent and should be treated with both surgical and therapy intervention. Surgical excision should be followed by strict voice rest (3-5 days) and immediate post-operative voice therapy aimed at reducing hard glottal onsets and pushed voicing (often a "confidential voice" is encouraged, page 90).

In some cases, small doses of Botox are injected at the time of surgery. These injections temporarily reduce laryngeal pressure by weakening adduction during phonation, thereby taking pressure off the vocal processes. (For more information on Botox, see page 62.)

# Contact Ulcers

### Presentation
This type of lesion presents as an ulceration on the medial surface of the arytenoid cartilage. Contact ulcers may be unilateral or bilateral with ulceration on one side and granulation tissue contralaterally from chronic irritation. They exhibit a ball and socket appearance—mass with concavity on the opposite side.

### Etiology

Contact ulcers are most often a result of vocal trauma or misuse, causing prolonged or forceful adduction of the vocal folds (e.g., coughing, yelling). They may also be precipitated or exacerbated by gastroesophageal reflux (GER). (For more information on GER, see pages 74-76.)

### Effects on vocal function and voice production

Contact ulcers may or may not affect the voice due to their posterior location on a non-vibratory or free margin of the vocal fold. If the voice is affected, the result is most often a harsh vocal quality with habitual glottal fry. The patient may report vocal fatigue and engage in chronic throat-clearing. Patients will frequently complain of laryngeal pain radiating to the ear on the ipsalateral side.

### Treatment

Contact ulcers (similar to granuloma) are often recurrent and should be treated with both surgical and therapeutic intervention. In some cases, small doses of Botox are used to reduce adduction. (For more information on Botox, see page 62.) Often, medication for GER is prescribed to reduce posterior laryngeal irritation.

## Reinke's Edema (also called *polypoid degeneration*)

### Presentation

Reinke's edema results from a collection of mucoid material within Reinke's space (see Figure 18, page 19). It may present unilaterally or bilaterally as diffuse vocal fold edema that is usually asymmetrical (one different from the other).

### Etiology

Smoking accounts for most all cases of Reinke's edema; however, it may also be associated with inflammation resulting from GER.

### Effects on vocal function and voice production

The voice is characteristically hoarse and diplophonic secondary to increased mass. This is often heard as a "smoker's voice." Sometimes cough and, in severe cases, stridor may accompany voice change.

### Treatment

Patients should be encouraged to stop smoking and GER medication is often prescribed. Surgical intervention to extract the fluid within Reinke's space is often performed; however, if smoking cessation does not occur, the edema will often reappear due to continued irritation. (Many surgeons will only perform the surgery if a patient has quit smoking.)

## Laryngeal Papilloma

### Presentation

Laryngeal papilloma is a benign collection of tumors of the epithelium with a wart-like appearance. These lesions can occur on the vocal folds, subglottally or supraglottally. Because papilloma lesions are viral in origin, they are highly recurrent (with periods of dormancy).

Papilloma lesions are often aggressive and resistant to treatment. The growths may compromise the airway and in severe cases require tracheostomy.

### Etiology
The cause of papilloma lesions is believed to be viral.

### Effects on vocal function and voice production
Epithelial invasion results in reduced vocal fold vibration and stiffness of the mucosa, resulting in severe hoarseness. An overgrowth of papilloma on the vocal folds can impact the glottal airway and result in stridor.

### Treatment
Treatment is surgical excision. However, given the generalized epithelial invasion and frequency of recurrence, repeated surgery may result in stiffness/scarring of the membranous cover, which may result in permanent hoarseness. Interferon treatment has also been used with varying degrees of success to eradicate the virus.

## Laryngeal Web

### Presentation
A laryngeal web is located at the anterior commissure and appears as an interconnecting membranous tissue band between the folds.

### Etiology
Webbing may be the result of a congenital malformation. Any trauma to the epithelium (e.g., surgical scarring) may result in the formation of an interconnecting web as the tissue heals.

### Effects on vocal function and voice production
This interconnection results in a tethering effect that restricts the amplitude of vibration and reduces the propagation of the mucosal wave. The resulting voice may have a raised pitch secondary to increased tension (tethering) of the vocal folds. In the case of larger webs, the glottal airway may be obstructed, resulting in stridor.

There is an increased risk for webbing to occur after bilateral surgical excision of lesions (e.g., Reinke's edema, papilloma). In some cases, the otolaryngologist may operate on one vocal fold at a time to allow for adequate healing prior to operating on the other vocal fold.

### Treatment
Surgical excision of the web is performed to free or separate the membranous edges of the vocal folds.

## Sulcus Vocalis (vocal fold scar)

### Presentation
A sulcus presents as a furrowing or "bowing" along the edge of the membranous vocal fold. It creates an asymmetric appearance of the vocal fold edge along the margin. Sulci are located within the superficial layer of the lamina propria (see Figure 18, page 19) and are made up of collagenous fibers, resulting in fibrotic/thickened epithelium.

### Etiology
Vocal fold trauma (e.g., abuse, intubation) and/or surgical healing may result in scarring of the epithelium.

### Effects on vocal function and voice production
Dysphonia varies depending on location and size of the segment affected and the degree of tethering. Since a scar/sulcus results in reduced vibration/impaired mucosal wave and glottal closure, the voice may have one or a combination of the following characteristics: breathiness, increased pitch, diplophonia, and harshness.

### Treatment
Scars resulting in greater degrees of dysphonia can severely affect the ability of the patient to communicate and/or function on the job. It may also impact his lifestyle. These scars may be treated surgically. Surgical treatments include injections (e.g., steroids) to "loosen" or soften the fibrosis and improve vibratory function of the vocal folds or augmentation to "fill-in" the furrowed area (e.g., collagen, autologous fat).

In some cases, the patient will be referred for voice therapy in an effort to restore vocal flexibility. Therapy tasks may include the following:

- pitch glides and scales—Use an /a/ or /m/ with increasing and decreasing pitches to "stretch" the vocal folds.
- trills—lip and tongue trills to encourage easy vibration
- improve resonance—nasal (pages 125-129) to focus the voice away from the larynx
- inflection/intonation exercises (pages 122-124) to improve vocal control

## Hyperkeratosis

### Presentation
Hyperkeratotic lesions originate on the epithelial level or deeper into the superficial lamina propria. They appear as abnormal tissue growths that are white, rough, plaque-like lesions with irregular margins on the mucosal surface of the vocal folds. They may present unilaterally or bilaterally. Hyperkeratosis may also present with cellular atypia/pre-malignant cellular growth.

### Etiology
Irritants to the larynx such as smoking, environmental pollutants, and gastroesophageal reflux (GER) may cause hyperkeratosis.

### Effects on vocal function and voice production
The surface of the vocal folds becomes thickened and results in a reduction of mucosal wave propagation, resulting in hoarseness and/or harshness of the voice.

### Treatment
Treatment includes biopsy of the lesion/lesions by an otolaryngologist with surgical or medical management as indicated. The patient should be counseled regarding potential irritants and their removal (e.g., quit smoking, wear a face mask if working in dusty or chemical environments).

## Leukoplakia and Erythroplakia

### Presentation
*Leukoplakia* presents as diffuse white, patchy lesions covering the vocal fold membrane. *Erythroplakia* presents as diffuse patchy, reddish lesions of the vocal fold membrane. These conditions may co-occur on the vocal folds.

### Etiology (same as hyperkeratosis, page 72)
Irritants to the larynx, such as smoking, environmental pollutants, and gastroesophageal reflux, (GER) may cause leukoplakia and/or erythroplakia.

Both conditions may extend to the subepithelial level and are often considered precancerous or pre-malignant. These conditions may represent carcinoma in situ (early, localized malignancy).

### Effects on vocal function and voice production
These conditions cause a diffuse, generalized thickening subepithelially, resulting in reduced vibration and, therefore, lowered pitch. The changes in the membrane surface properties may result in hoarseness and possibly reduced volume.

### Treatment
Treatment includes biopsy of the lesion/lesions by an otolaryngologist with surgical or medical management as indicated. The patient should be counseled regarding potential irritants and their removal (e.g., quit smoking, wear a face mask if working in dusty or chemical environments).

## Cancer

Cancerous lesions may occur at many places within the oral cavity, pharynx, larynx, and upper airway, and therefore, have significant and often life-altering effects on the voice and oral communication. Laryngeal cancer is listed within this chapter as an organic pathology; however, review of its presentation, treatment, and management requires more detailed explanation. Chapter 5, pages 140-162, will cover head and neck cancers and vocal rehabilitation.

# Gastro-Esophageal Reflux Disease (GERD)

Literature has reported findings of gastro-esophageal reflux (GER) as a significant contributing factor in hoarseness and the development of vocal pathologies (Koufman et al. 1996; Toohill & Kuhn 1997). It has been reported that approximately half the patients with voice and/or laryngeal disorders have GER as a causative agent (Koufman & Cummings 1995).

Abbreviations used in this section:
    GERD—gastro-esophageal reflux disease
    GER—gastro-esophageal reflux
    LPR—laryngo-pharyngeal reflux, reflux laryngitis

## BACKGROUND INFORMATION

LPR may be called *atypical* or *extra-esophageal reflux* because it describes the spillage of stomach acid out of the esophagus and onto the posterior portion of the larynx. Acid coming into contact with the laryngeal structures may cause inflammation and/or tissue change. Subtle laryngeal changes resulting from LPR can be detected upon visualization performed by the SLP or ENT. These changes include pachyderma (thickening or hypertrophy of tissue), erythema (redness), and edema (swelling), most often involving the posterior larynx. Laryngeal irritation and tissue changes secondary to LPR/GER can lead to organic pathologies including the following:

- reflux laryngitis (pages 65-66)
- granuloma (page 69)
- contact ulcers (pages 69-70)
- Reinke's edema/polypoid degeneration (page 70)
- leukoplakia/erythroplakia (page 73)
- carcinoma (pages 140-162)
- subglottic stenosis (narrowing of the upper airway)

Laryngeal irritation resulting from LPR may also be a contributory factor in hyperfunctional disorders. For example, if laryngeal edema or irritation results in vibratory changes, the patient may compensate with excessive strain or tension during phonation.

## SYMPTOMS

It is possible for a patient to have LPR/GER without experiencing "heartburn." Unlike the esophagus, the larynx does not have protective mechanisms against acidity, and therefore patients may not exhibit symptoms of esophagitis (esophageal irritation/heartburn). Laryngeal symptoms may include the following:

- hoarseness/dysphonia
- chronic throat clearing
- globus sensation (lump in throat)
- cough
- laryngeal soreness/pain
- dysphagia and/or odynophagia (pain upon swallowing)
- paroxysmal laryngospasm (sudden onset of laryngeal spasm)

74

## TREATMENT

Treatment of GER/LPR should include both medication and changes in diet and lifestyle. In cases of severe persistent GER resistant to pharmacologic treatment, patients may require surgical intervention. Fundoplication (Nissen fundoplication) is often the surgical treatment of choice. In essence, this procedure involves a "wrap" of the stomach around the lower portion of the esophagus to tighten the lower esophageal sphincter (LES) and reduce the backflow of stomach contents/acid into the esophagus.

## Medications

The most frequently prescribed drug classes for LPR/GER include proton pump inhibitors (PPI) and H2 antagonists. Both of these drug classes essentially inhibit or reduce the amount of acid that is produced and is present in the gastrointestinal tract. Prescription medications play a crucial role in controlling reflux to reduce laryngeal inflammation.

Recent literature (Shaw et al. 1996, Shaw & Searl 1997) has reported improved laryngeal healing with the use of PPIs (lanzoprezole/omeprazole). These medications include brand names such as Prilosec, Nexium, Prevacid, Aciphex, and Protonix. Patients may take these medications as prescribed by their physicians for a period of six weeks to three months prior to reporting an improvement in laryngeal symptoms. The patient should have a follow-up visit with his physician to assess any change in laryngeal inflammation or reduction of organic pathology after approximately 12 weeks of pharmacologic treatment.

## Dietary Modifications

Modification to a patient's diet can also be an effective way to control LPR/GER. Diet recommendations include a bland diet, with reduction in caffeine, citrus, alcoholic, and carbonated beverages. Foods with high acid content, such as tomato-based products or spicy foods, should be consumed in moderation. Foods containing mint or menthol should also be limited, including breath mints and throat lozenges. Other foods to avoid include onions, fatty foods, and chocolate. (See handout on page 76.)

## Lifestyle Modifications

In addition to dietary changes, various lifestyle changes can help decrease reflux symptoms. For example, elevate the head of the patient's bed with bricks or blocks (approximately four to six inches) under the headboard or use a wedge pillow to decrease reflux when lying down. Elevating the head by using multiple head pillows is not effective because it causes the torso to bend, creating increased visceral pressure. Patients should also avoid eating at least one to two hours before bedtime. Other modifications include not overeating and avoidance of tight or constrictive clothing such as belts or girdles. Patients should also attempt to lose any excess weight. Incorporating exercise into a patient's daily schedule can also help reduce stress, another contributory factor to GER. (See handout on page 76.)

# LPR/GERD Handout

Laryngopharyngeal Reflux (LPR) occurs when stomach acid redirects into the larynx (voice box) and pharynx (throat). Many patients exhibiting gastric reflux into the larynx may or may not report heartburn or indigestion.

You may experience one or more of the following symptoms associated with LPR/GER:

- cough
- throat-clearing
- feeling of something "caught" in your throat
- hoarseness
- sore throat
- difficulty swallowing
- pain or discomfort when you swallow
- bitter or acidic taste in your mouth

In addition to taking medication, which may be prescribed by your physician, it is important to follow the precautions listed below:

**Foods to Avoid**

| | |
|---|---|
| carbonated beverages | chocolate |
| caffeine | mint/menthol |
| onions | spicy foods/hot sauce |
| citrus fruits/juices | tomato-based foods (including salsa) |
| alcohol | |

**Lifestyle Modifications**

- Stop smoking.
- Elevate the head of your bed four to six inches. (Do not just use pillows—elevate your torso, too.)
- Lose any excess weight.
- Avoid tight or restrictive clothing.
- Exercise, but avoid weight lifting.
- Avoid eating one to two hours before bedtime.
- Avoid overeating.
- Decrease stress.

76

# Neurological Conditions Affecting the Voice

"Complex functions necessary for normal voice function require coordinated interactions among multiple body systems. Neurologic dysfunction that impairs control of these interactions commonly causes voice dysfunction." (Sataloff et al. 1997)

There are many neurological conditions that have an effect on the voice and/or speech production. It is important for the SLP to have a working knowledge of neuroanatomy, motor control of speech function, and disorders. The identification and treatment of motor speech disorders such as the types of dysarthria discussed in this section should be researched separately as they are outside the focus of this book (e.g., Duffy 1995).

This section will highlight disorders that are commonly associated with voice change, organized by site of lesion in an effort to tie the voice disorder to motor speech characteristics that often co-exist.

## UPPER MOTOR NEURON (UMN) LESIONS (result in spastic or hyper-reactive reflexes)

### Pseudobulbar palsy

**Etiology**
Pseudobulbar palsy may result from a cerebral vascular accident (CVA), head trauma, tumor, infection, or inflammatory or metabolic disease process.

**Effects on speech and voice production**
The resulting speech deficit is characterized as spastic dysarthria. Speech therapy should focus on articulation and precision of consonant production.

Vocal characteristics associated with pseudobulbar palsy may include a harsh or strained-strangled voice with lowered pitch, monoloudness, and hypernasality. Patients may also experience pitch breaks and inappropriate stress/prosody.

**Treatment**

*Respiratory control of voicing*
- breath support and control of airflow (pages 108-109)
- phrasing practice (page 110)
- sentences of increased length (page 111)

*Rate, prosody, and pitch variation*
- intonation practice (pages 124-126)

*Reduction of laryngeal hyperfunction/strain*
- easy onset practice (pages 121-123)
- continuous voicing practice (page 117)

### LOWER MOTOR NEURON (LMN) LESIONS (result in flaccid or hypotonic muscles)
- Bulbar palsy
- Myasthenia Gravis

## Bulbar palsy

### Etiology
Bulbar palsy may result from brainstem CVA, viral infection, tumor, or trauma to the cranial nerves (motor units).

### Effects on speech and voice production
The resulting speech deficit is characterized as *flaccid dysarthria*. Speech therapy should focus on oral (lingual/labial) strengthening and articulatory precision.

Vocal characteristics associated with bulbar palsy include a breathy/weak vocal quality with any combination of the following: hypernasality, monotone, monoloudness, and use of short phrases. There is a possibility of vocal fold paresis/paralysis that may be bilateral or unilateral, causing inspiratory stridor (noise on inhalation).

### Treatment

*Improved respiratory support for voicing*
- diaphragmatic breathing (page 104)
- breath support and control of airflow (pages 105-106)
- phrasing practice (pages 107)
- sentences of increased length (page 108)

*Increasing volume and variations of loudness*
- use of background noise to encourage use of louder speech
- compare soft and loud productions

*Improved adduction/hypofunction*
- adduction exercises (pages 101-102)
- pitch glides for improved medial closure—Have the patient produce a low-pitched and then high-pitched hum using /a/ or /i/.
- pitch scales from lower to higher pitches (e.g., sing a scale).

## Myasthenia Gravis

### Etiology
Myasthenia Gravis may result from brainstem CVA, viral infection, tumor, or trauma to the cranial nerves (motor units).

### Effects on speech and voice production

The resulting speech deficit is characterized as flaccid dysarthria. Speech therapy should focus on oral (lingual/labial) strengthening and articulatory precision.

The vocal characteristic associated with myasthenia gravis is voice deterioration over time with extended use. The voice becomes increasingly breathy and decreases in volume during speaking, due to muscle fatigue and poor breath support/respiratory weakness. Patients often experience hypernasalisty and nasal emission.

### Treatment

Hyperadduction techniques and respiratory support
- use of "pushed" or "forced" phonation
- phrasing (page 107)

Palatal lifts are used to improve velar closure and reduce hypernasality.

Medical management, including hormone and pharmacologic treatments (pyridostigmine/Mestinon) are effective at controlling the symptoms of muscle weakness seen with myasthenia gravis.

## MIXED UMN/LMN LESIONS (result in weak muscles with hyperactive reflexes or spasticity)

# ALS (amyotrophic lateral sclerosis or Lou Gehrig's disease)

### Etiology

The etiology of ALS is unknown. ALS results in a progressive degeneration of the motor neurons of the UMN and LMN tracts, resulting in symptoms of both spasticity and muscle weakness.

### Effects on speech and voice production

The resulting speech deficit includes any combination of those seen in spastic or flaccid dysarthria. Speech therapy focuses on the training for use of an alternative communication device.

Vocal characteristics associated with ALS may include symptoms of both pseudobulbar and bulbar palsy (e.g., harshness, strain, poor vocal adduction resulting in breathiness and reduced phrase length, changes in rate, lowered pitch, hypernasality, and often a "wet" vocal quality).

### Treatment

Palatal lifts have been used in earlier stages of the disease process to improve nasality. Direct treatment is not typically advocated due to the rapidly progressing effects on voice and speech. Family education and counseling regarding the loss of communication and use of alternative devices is recommended.

**BASAL GANGLIA (BG) LESIONS** (affect the integration and control of complex movements and the inhibition of involuntary movement, resulting in dyskinesia)

- Parkinson's Disease
- Huntington's Chorea
- Dystonias
    Spasmodic Dysphonia
    Essential Tremor
    Multiple Sclerosis

Dyskinetic movements may be of two types:
**Hypokinetic**: reduction of movement; results in rigidity
**Hyperkinetic**: increase in movement; results in spasticity or tremor

## Parkinson's Disease

**Etiology**
The etiology of Parkinson's Disease is unknown. It is a degenerative condition of the substantia nigra and consequently chemical depletion of the neural transmitter dopamine carrying signals for initiation of voluntary movement. This depletion results in muscular rigidity, resting tremor, difficulty with movement initiation (bradykinesia), and slowness of voluntary movement.

**Effects on speech and voice production**
Speech exhibits a hypokinetic dysarthria. Speech therapy should focus on articulatory precision, rate, and prosodic variation.

Vocal characteristics associated with Parkinson's disease include hoarseness, breathiness, vocal tremor, monopitch, and reduced volume.

Note: Vocal folds may present with bowing upon visualization such as with mirror examination and/or laryngoscopy.

**Treatment**
Medications include dopaminergic drugs (Sinemet), Levadopa, and dopamine agonists, which serve to replace lost dopamine and resulting in decreased rigidity and increased movment. Anticholinergic drugs are sometimes used in early stages to control resting tremors.

The most well recognized formal treatment approach for patients with Parkinson's disease is the Lee Silverman Voice Treatment (LSVT) method. Efficacy studies (Ramig et al. 1994, Ramig 1995) have found LSVT to be effective at improving loudness and pitch variability as well as overall intelligibility.

Note: Training in LSVT technique is highly recommended for clinical efficacy. The following information is a brief overview of the principles of this treatment approach; however, continuing education in the utilization of the proposed protocol is strongly suggested.

*Principles of LSVT*

Therapy is performed four times a week for four weeks.

Therapy is designed to do the following:

1. increase vocal fold adduction
2. improve respiratory support
3. increase pitch range

The above parameters are targeted through:

- use of increased phonatory effort and vocal fold adduction through the use of "loud speech"—THINK LOUD
- systematic use of prolonged vowels with adduction exercises (pages 101-102)
- use of pitch glides
- progression from simple to complex speech drills (words, sentences, and/or paragraphs)

# Huntington's Chorea

### Etiology

Huntington's Chorea is an inherited (autosomal dominant), progressive disease, that results in the loss of neurons from the cerebral cortex, caudate nucleus, and palladium, which, in turn, results in involuntary movements that are irregular or spasmodic. These abrupt, purposeless movements of the head, neck, or limbs are termed *choreaform movements*.

### Effects on speech and voice production

The resulting speech deficit is a hyperkinetic dysarthria. Speech therapy is often not initiated secondary to the progressive loss of movement.

Vocal characteristics associated with Huntington's Chorea include harshness, strained-strangled quality, intermittent breathiness, and hypernasality. Pitch is most often lowered with pitch breaks and/or aphonic breaks. Poor respiratory support with poorly coordinated breathing results in sudden bursts of loudness.

### Treatment

A brief course of therapy may be implemented to teach compensatory/maintenance strategies, such as reduced rate and shorter phrase length. However, given the progressive decline in speech and voice, family counseling regarding communication is recommended.

Pharmacologic treatment using medications that reduce the dopamine effects on the body (e.g., Haldol, Klonopin, Thorazine) serve to reduce involuntary movements, such as tics.

## Dystonia

Dystonia is another form of hyperkinesia. It affects primarily the trunk, neck, and proximal part of the limbs, resulting in poor coordination of voluntary movements.

### Etiology
The etiology of dystonia may include vascular lesions, encephalitis, and degenerative neuron disease processes.

Spasmodic dysphonia has been previously described as a type of focal dystonia (page 61). However other forms of dystonia (e.g., essential tremor, torticollis, facial spasms) may accompany SD. The most common accompanying dystonia is Meige syndrome. Meige syndrome is an oromandibular dystonia resulting in dyskinesia of the eyelids, face, and tongue.

Dystonias are often treated with anticholoinergics such as Parsidol, resulting in improved control over movements with reduced tremor.

## Essential Tremor (often called *familial tremor* or *senile tremor*)

### Etiology
Essential tremor is a disorder of the central nervous system (CNS) with localization not well understood.

Essential tremor appears to be associated with aging. Tremor may or may not be absent during rest (resting tremor). Typically the tremor appears during maintenance of a fixed posture/ position against gravity or during active movement. Essential tremor may result in tremor of the head, tongue, and palate as well as the hands and arms.

### Effects on speech and voice production
The resulting speech deficits range from a slight disorder in articulation to severe articulatory breakdown with reduced intelligibility, depending on the degree of tremor affecting the jaw and tongue. Speech therapy focuses on slowed rate and articulatory precision.

Vocal characteristics associated with tremor include low pitch with pitch breaks (most observable during sustained vowel production), intermittent strained quality, and a monotonous quality. Vocal tremor occurs from tremor of both the intrinsic and extrinsic laryngeal muscles.

Differential diagnosis of spasmodic dysphonia (SD) vs. essential tremor may be difficult. Essential tremor results in more regular or rhythmic oscillations in pitch and loudness, whereas SD results in irregular vocal patterns and complete phonatory/vocal arrests.

### Treatment

Voice therapy focuses on contrasting tension vs. relaxation.
- contrast pushed phonation/hyperadduction vs. breathiness
- chewing exercises (page 92)
- yawn-sigh technique (page 92)

Note: Therapy is most often used to relax compensatory behaviors rather than direct treatment of the tremor.

Medications include Inderal (beta blocker), which has been shown to reduce the amplitude of the tremors.

## Multiple Sclerosis (MS)

### Etiology
The etiology of MS is unknown but may be viral in nature.

MS is a disease process that causes demyelination (loss of the myelin cover) of neural axons within white matter. Lesions affect the entire CNS and occasionally peripheral nervous systems.

### Effects on speech and voice production
The resulting speech deficit is a mixed spastic-ataxic dysarthria. Although many patients do not experience articulatory breakdowns, speech may be reduced in rate with impaired prosody. Speech therapy should focus on improved prosody and phrasing.

Vocal characteristics associated with MS include poor control of volume and pitch, breathiness, poor breath support, and hypernasality.

### Treatment

*Improving breathing and breath support*
- diaphragmatic breathing (page 104)
- airflow control techniques (pages 105-106)
- phrasing (page 107)
- sentence of increasing length (page 108)

*Increasing vocal hyperfunction/adduction and loudness*
- adduction exercises (pages 101-102)
- use of increased loudness with background noise
- amplification often recommended

*Improving pitch control*
- pitch glides on vowels (/a/ and /i/) from low to high pitch.
- intonation practice (pages 122-124)

Medications include adrenal corticosteroids that reduce the duration of acute exacerbations and muscle relaxants to reduce spasticity.

# Additional Medical Conditions That May Affect Vocal Quality

During the collection of case/medical history, SLPs should have a cursory knowledge of conditions that may have negative effects on the voice and laryngeal mucosa. The following disorders have documented negative effects on the larynx and may result in changes in vocal quality, including hoarseness, lowered pitch, and reduced pitch range.

## INFLAMMATORY DISEASES AFFECTING THE LARYNX

The following disorders cause inflammation and erythema (swelling) of tissues, mucous membranes, and/or joints. As a result, the voice may exhibit hoarseness, reduced pitch, and stiffness/restriction of range. These disorders include the following:

- allergic/hypersensitivity reactions such as angioedema and Stephen-Johnson syndrome
- autoimmune disorders such as rheumatoid arthritis, lupus, pemphagoid, polycondritis, and Sjogren's syndrome

## ENDOCRINE DISORDERS AND HORMONAL CHANGES

Disturbance in endocrine and hormone levels can result in edema or fluid changes in the laryngeal mucosa. This often results in a reduction in pitch. These disorders include the following:

- endocrine disorders, such as Cushing's syndrome and thyroid disorders/diseases such as Hashimoto's (hypothyroidism)
- hormonal changes, such as gonadal disorders in males and menses and pregnancy in females

# 4 • TREATMENT

When treating patients with voice disorders, the clinician must keep current with the development of new techniques, standards of care, and evidence-based practice models. The efficacy of voice therapy has been widely studied and reported in the literature. ASHA (2005) provides a comprehensive review of the literature supporting the use of voice therapy in the management of patients with vocal pathology and voice disorders.

The following chapter has been designed to review various treatment approaches and provide treatment tasks and stimulus items to target a variety of vocal behaviors. Included are examples of clinical cues for use within the sessions to facilitate the desired production, and may be photocopied for patients to use during out-of-clinic practice. The sections included within the chapter cover the following areas:

- Vocal Hygiene
- Voice Therapy Theories and Approaches
- Therapy Exercises/Tasks
  Physical Exercises
  Respiration/Airflow
  Phonation
  Resonance (oral and nasal)

## Vocal Hygiene

Vocal hygiene encompasses many parameters related to vocal health. These areas may include modifications in lifestyle or behaviors. It is crucial to include a vocal hygiene component to every voice therapy treatment plan in order to optimize success in therapy. It is important to thoroughly assess the patient's risk factors and provide suggestions for remediation of these vocally "unhygienic" behaviors. However, it is also important to remember that it is often not feasible for patients to completely change their lifestyles in order to be vocally hygienic. Therefore, the information that follows should be presented in moderation.

Vocal hygiene can be described as three components:

- vocal health
- vocal abuse
- vocal misuse

### VOCAL HEALTH

Prior to initiating voice therapy, it is important to evaluate the patient's lifestyle and assess it for factors that may have an impact on her voice. Hydration has a significant effect on the voice and can be beneficial in facilitating a reduction in irritation to the vocal fold tissues. It is recommended that all patients increase water intake, both systemically and environmentally. This can be accomplished by consuming at least eight 8-ounce glasses of water per day and using a cool-mist humidifier. Increased hydration will also decrease the viscosity of mucous that may collect on the vocal folds. Breathing through the nose rather than the mouth will also moisten the air as the patient inhales.

Since caffeine is a diuretic, it is important to limit the consumption of products that contain high levels of caffeine, including coffee, tea, chocolate, and some carbonated beverages. In addition to decreasing caffeine intake, other dietary modifications may also be necessary in order to promote good vocal hygiene.  For patients with a history of gastroesophageal reflux disease (GERD), dietary modifications may be necessary in addition to compliance with prescribed medications.  (See pages 74-76 for GERD recommendations.)

Any smoking and use of inhalers should also be reduced and, if possible, eliminated in order to reduce irritation or change in the composition of vocal fold tissues.  Patients should be strongly encouraged to discontinue smoking in order to improve vocal hygiene and reduce the risk for developing laryngeal pathologies.  The environments in which the patient spends most of her time should also be assessed for potential environmental irritants, including excessive dust, airborne chemicals, and allergens.

It is important to have the patient provide a current list of all medications she is taking.  You should be familiar with medications or classes of medications that have an effect on the voice (hoarseness, dryness, cough).  These medications include inhaled steroids, antihistamines, ace-inhibitors, and diuretics.  Certain psychotropic medications (depressants and stimulants) may also have an effect on speech and/or voice.  (See page 41 for a list of medications and their effects on voice/speech.)  Of course, any modification in prescription medications must be made by a physician.

Help patients become aware of characteristics that make an environment vocally unhygienic and encourage them to choose environments that optimize vocal hygiene.  For example, talk about taking into consideration the acoustic properties of a room as well as the distance from speakers to listeners.  Encourage them to control environmental factors by selecting seating in restaurants away from increased noise (kitchen area, door, bar); decreasing background noise by turning down the television, radio, air conditioner; and using air filters in smoky or dust-filled places.  Amplification options should be explored for speaking professionals such as lecturers and teachers.  (See Classroom Amplification, page 167.)

## Summary of Recommendations for Vocal Health

Discuss the following recommendations with patients to improve their vocal health.

- Increase hydration and humidification.
- Reduce/eliminate caffeine.
- GERD/reflux precautions:  dietary modifications and medical management (pages 74-76)
- Reduce/eliminate smoking.
- Identify medications that may have side effects including hoarseness and/or cough (page 41).
- Encourage patients to discuss use of prescription inhalers with physician (if cause hoarseness).
- Assess environment for airborne irritants (wear mask if necessary).
- Reduce exposure to allergens.
- Assess acoustic properties of a room and modify as needed.
- Use amplification during periods of extended projected voice use (public speaking).

*The Vocal Hygiene Patient Questionnaire* (page 87) and *Vocal Hygiene Modification List* (page 88) provide information regarding lifestyle modifications for a healthy voice.

# Vocal Hygiene Patient Questionnaire

Name _____ Date _____

## Vocal Hygiene

Caffeine intake (glasses/cups per day of coffee, soda, tea, chocolate) _____

Water intake (8-oz. glasses per day) _____

Alcohol intake (drinks per week) _____

Smoking history (packs per day, year quit) _____

Current medications _____

Allergies _____

Occupation _____

Hours per day spent talking _____

Work environment (noise level, exposure to irritants) _____

## Vocal Abuse

| | | | | |
|---|---|---|---|---|
| Do you clear your throat frequently? | Yes | No | Sometimes | Explain. _____ |
| Do you cough? | Yes | No | Sometimes | Is it productive? _____ |
| Do you talk excessively? | Yes | No | Sometimes | Explain. _____ |
| Do you scream/yell? | Yes | No | Sometimes | Explain. _____ |
| Do you imitate noises? | Yes | No | Sometimes | Explain. _____ |
| Do you talk loudly? | Yes | No | Sometimes | Explain. _____ |
| Do you grunt while exercising? | Yes | No | Sometimes | Explain. _____ |

## Vocal Misuse

| | | | | |
|---|---|---|---|---|
| Do you talk when stressed? | Yes | No | Sometimes | Frequency? _____ |
| Do you talk when tired? | Yes | No | Sometimes | Frequency? _____ |
| Do you use a low/high pitch? | Yes | No | Sometimes | Frequency? _____ |
| Do you use character voices? | Yes | No | Sometimes | Frequency? _____ |
| Do you talk when you have a cold/ upper respiratory infection? | Yes | No | Sometimes | Frequency? _____ |

# Vocal Hygiene Modification List

Many factors impact the health and performance of the voice, but some modifications are relatively easy to incorporate into a daily lifestyle. Below is a list of factors that may impact vocal hygiene and lifestyle modifications for each one.

| Factors | Modifications |
|---|---|
| Complaint of dryness/thick secretions | Increase water intake. |
| | Use humidification (may be contraindicated for patients with mold allergies). |
| | Use throat lozenges (not mint/menthol). |
| | Decrease caffeine intake. |
| | Decrease the use of antihistamines (if approved by a physician). |
| | Breathe through the nose. |
| | Check medications for side effects. |
| | Possible allergy testing if other allergy symptoms are present (e.g., itchy eyes, post-nasal drip) |
| | If severe, use prescription or nonprescription saliva-producing agents (e.g., Mouth-Kote, Salagen). |
| Excessive screaming or yelling/loud speaking environments | Use nonverbal methods to gain attention (e.g., whistles, hand wave). |
| | Relocate/move in order to speak face-to-face with someone. |
| | Use amplification. |
| | Reduce background noise (e.g., TV, radio, machinery). |
| Complaint of vocal fatigue | Use vocal warm-ups if performing. |
| | Reduce "talk time." |
| | Incorporate "voice rest" into daily schedule. |
| Excessive throat clearing/coughing | GER management (pages 74-76) |
| | Engage in a "silent cough." |
| | Reduce/eliminate smoking. |
| | Check medications for side effects. |
| | Assess swallowing/secretion management. |

## VOCAL ABUSE

Vocal abuse includes behaviors that place the vocal folds at risk for damage/irritation. In many instances, factors that can influence the presence of vocally abusive behaviors may include work environment, characteristics of personal expression, and habitual behaviors. Excessive and prolonged voice use is a primary factor when identifying or evaluating vocal abuse. Nonspeech behaviors like excessive throat-clearing or coughing and imitating sounds (e.g., motors, animal noises) are also considered vocally-abusive

Patients who engage in excessive voice use, especially in environments that are loud, are at a higher risk to develop a vocal pathology. When speaking in loud environments or large spaces, individuals generally use increased volume levels and sometimes have the tendency to yell or shout.

Many professions place patients at a higher risk for vocal abuse due to work settings and vocal demands. These occupations may include teaching, coaching, customer service/sales representatives, ministering, counseling, and frequent public speaking. (See page 133 for speaking recommendations.)

While producing abusive behaviors, the vocal folds hit each other/adduct with excessive force (glottal attack). Increased volume also requires tight adduction of the vocal folds and increased subglottic air pressures. These vocal behaviors and hyperfunction within the system create an increased risk for irritation to vocal fold tissues and potential mucosal changes.

### Examples of Vocal Abuse

- increased volume
- prolonged talking
- excessive throat-clearing or coughing
- yelling, screaming, or shouting
- excessive laughing or crying
- imitation of animal/mechanical sounds
- grunting during exercise/weight lifting

## VOCAL MISUSE

Vocal misuse, in comparison to vocal abuse, is identified as improper use of one's voice. This may include speaking in a less than optimal pitch or volume. In addition to pitch and volume, vocal misuse can occur from speaking in long utterances without adequate breath support. This may result from an increased rate of speech or from not stopping "for air" when talking. This type of behavior will often result in strain and/or vocal fatigue. Altered prosody is often present in patients with vocal misuse.

In order to assess these behaviors and to facilitate voice production that is within normal limits for age and gender, it is important to use both perceptual/subjective and objective measurements. See Chapter 2, pages 20-36, for behavioral, acoustic, and aerodynamic assessment tools.

Patients at higher risk for voice misuse include customer service employees or telemarketers who engage in extended speaking periods of repetitive material, singers who attempt to sing outside of their "natural" ranges, and actors/actresses who frequently produce a variety of character voices.

Talking during an upper respiratory infection may also contribute to vocal misuse due to the need to engage compensatory forced phonation strategies in order to get enough volume to be heard by others. It is important to remember not to talk "through" a cold or laryngitis!

## Examples of Voice Misuse

- Using a pitch that is too high/low for age and gender
- Inadequate use of airflow/breath support
- Decreased intonation/pitch variation
- Talking through an upper respiratory infection or cold
- Singing outside of one's "natural" range  (See pages 134-135 for singing terminology and guidelines.)
- Production of character voices
- Speaking when under stress or tired

# Theories and Approaches

The efficacy of many voice therapy techniques has been challenged in the literature (Pannbacker 1998). The following approaches have been demonstrated as effective for particular voice disorders. Although certain tasks are suggested in Chapter 3 as a starting point, therapy techniques should be tailored to the disorder and needs of each individual patient and used by skilled clinicians. A "blanket prescription" of tasks and/or exercises cannot and should not be used based on a diagnosis alone.

It is also important to emphasize that the vocal quality the patient produces during many of these therapeutic exercises is often not the end result of therapy. The exercises are used to promote a certain vocal quality to be later shaped into everyday, habitual voice use.

## CONFIDENTIAL VOICE THERAPY

This technique is also called *breathy phonation*. It is useful in hyperfunctional disorders (e.g., vocal fold nodules) and/or traumatic injuries to the voice (e.g., traumatic laryngitis). The premise is that the vocal folds are slightly open during phonation (Colton & Casper 1995).

Instruct the patient to use a soft voice (reduced loudness) as if speaking confidentially. This behavior reduces hyperfunction and focuses awareness on expiratory airflow to produce the voice.

## RESONANT VOICE THERAPY

This technique is also referred to as the *Lessac technique*. It is used in the treatment of functional voice disorders, hyperfunctional pathologies, and vocal fold atrophy or paresis. The technique emphasizes the sensation and placement of oral resonance, often at the anterior palate. It uses a forward focus to establish a strong, clear, resonant tone while promoting a relaxed laryngeal posture.

Therapy uses a series of hierarchical tasks moving from nasal to non-nasal consonants with variation in pitch and loudness to stimuli of increasing length and finally into conversational voice use (Verdolini 1998). Tasks with nasal onsets are provided on pages 127-129.

## VOCAL FUNCTION EXERCISES

This technique is used for a variety of hyper- and hypofunctional disorders and aids in strengthening and increasing flexibility of the laryngeal muscles. It is based on vocal physiology and the use of physical exercise techniques with a targeted muscle group.

This approach uses a series of pitch exercises with glides and scales with sustained vowels and target word productions. A four-step protocol has been developed for clinical use (Stemple et al. 1995).

## LARYNGEAL MASSAGE

This technique is used primarily to reduce musculoskeletal tension in hyperfunctional voice disorders. It involves direct palpation of the patient's laryngeal area.

Digital massage of the hyoid bone and thyroid cartilage is used with the addition of voice production (hum or prolonged vowel), moving into increasing length of utterances while reinforcing improvements in vocal quality. The massage is then gradually withdrawn. Explanation of this technique and variation in techniques are offered by Aronson (1985) and Morrison & Rammage (1993).

## ACCENT METHOD

This technique has been used in many types of voice disorders as it focuses on multiple parameters, including breathing, airflow, and relaxation/tension with rhythmic movements of the body and works toward the addition of vocal practice.

Initial instruction focuses on awareness of abdominal muscles and a rhythmic breathing pattern alternating contraction and release. Phonation is added using rhythmic syllable production and materials such as nursery rhymes in which the rhythm and pitch are accentuated. Use of body movements is added to release tension and then later withdrawn once the rhythmic breathing and vocal production is established (Smith & Thyme 1976).

## LEE SILVERMAN VOICE TREATMENT (LSVT)

LSVT has gained recognition in the literature as a therapeutic approach effective at targeting hypofunctional vocal quality as in Parkinson's disease (Ramig 1995).

Patients are instructed to use increased phonatory effort and increased vocal fold adduction through the use of "loud speech." Treatment also incorporates the use of adduction exercise, prolonged vowels, and pitch glides. (See pages 80-81 for a more detailed explanation of treatment of dysphonia associated with Parkinson's.)

## OTHER TECHNIQUES

Other facilitative techniques used in voice therapy have been reported in the literature as effective in targeting a desired vocal effect (Boone & McFarlane 2000, Casper & Murry 2000).

The following is a list of the most commonly used voice therapy techniques with a brief description of each:

- Auditory feedback—may be immediate or delayed; with or without amplification

- Auditory masking—delivery of masking noise under headphones that inhibits the patient's ability to self-monitor vocal quality

- Chant talk—use of one continuous tone through many connected syllables using an increased pitch and prolonged vowels

- Chewing (Froeschels chewing)—use of exaggerated rotary (lateral and vertical) chewing during phonation and release of jaw/mandibular tension

- Ingressive phonation—phonation on inspiration to produce a "stridorous" vocal quality and then immediate release to phonation on exhalation

- Open mouth—use of an open-mouthed posture to improve oral resonance and increase the feeling of space in the oral cavity during phonation

- Yawn-sigh—use of a yawn to open the oropharyngeal space and lower the larynx (use of a visual cue such as "open the back of your throat to fit a golf ball" will often promote a yawn posture). On the exhalation phase of the yawn, the patient produces a relaxed vocal sigh.

## ADDRESSING GLOTTAL FRY

There is significant controversy in the literature whether "to treat or not to treat." Glottal fry is considered one of the vocal registers (pulse register) and often considered part of "normal" vocal production. However, persistent or habitual use of glottal fry is considered to be hyperfunctional and causes increased tension in the larynx. It is my belief and experience that reduction of the use of glottal fry improves vocal quality and reduces laryngeal tension.

The following discussion outlines the pros and cons of the use of this vocal register. You may wish to address these in therapy.

*Clinical note*:   Glottal fry is most often heard at the end of a sentence or phrase as both pitch and intensity drop off.

| PROS | CONS |
|---|---|
| The production of "true" glottal fry involves the use of relaxed laryngeal posture/lax vocal folds with just enough subglottic air pressure needed to generate voicing. It has been described as "phonating quietly at the lowest possible pitch" (Zemlin 1998). | The pulse register of glottal fry is produced at the bottom of the pitch range and therefore is very inflexible. Production of glottal fry involves a longer closed phase of vibration and requires tightly adducted vocal folds with lax or flaccid vibratory margins. Although glottal fry requires lower airflow, there is a significant reduction in energy over time; therefore, it is difficult to achieve volume without increased tension. Habitual use of glottal fry is considered hyperfunctional and often results in vocal fatigue. |

## OPTIMAL PITCH

It has been both documented and challenged in the literature that optimal speaking pitch falls at a specific place within the total pitch range (25-35% the way up the total range.) (See Chapter 2, page 26, for frequency norms.) As a result, there is much controversy as to whether the concept of "an optimal pitch" should be directly addressed in therapy by having the patient "speak higher" or "speak lower." The controversy lies in the fact that many other parameters have an effect on the perception of pitch, such as loudness, dysphonia, or air escape (breathiness).

During the evaluation process, both objective testing and subjective/perceptual judgments regarding pitch should be considered. Objective measures (see jitter/perturbation measures, page 27) provide you with information regarding the stability of the vibration of the vocal folds at various frequencies/pitches. Keep in mind that an inappropriate pitch level may be either the cause or result of a voice disorder or pathology. For example, speaking or singing for prolonged periods of time at an unnatural or forced pitch may contribute to the development of vocal fold nodules. The presence of nodules may also result in a lowered vocal pitch or a reduced pitch range.

Subjective impressions during speaking and the use of probe techniques (e.g., vegetative phonation) are helpful in determining if a patient is using an appropriate pitch level during habitual speech Using vegetative tasks (e.g., sigh, relaxed hum) may elicit a vocal tone that is different from the patient's speaking voice. This difference may suggest a behavioral or functional component (e.g., tension, habitual glottal fry), resulting in a pitch change that may be addressed in therapy.

Therefore, it is the combined physiological and functional assessment of pitch that should assist you in formulating behavioral objectives to address during therapy. Think of addressing "optimal pitch" by providing therapy tasks that focus on establishing the clearest, most resonant vocal tone with the least amount of laryngeal effort. This approach should elicit stability of vocal fold vibration and consequently a more appropriate pitch.

# Therapy Exercises/Tasks

The following pages cover activities and materials to use in therapy to target specified voice goals. These goals should be determined based on the disorder being treated (diagnosis), the information gathered from the evaluation process, on-going assessment (functioning), and behavior observed (symptoms). Any additional patient complaints should also be addressed.

*Example*:

The patient is diagnosed with vocal fold paralysis (diagnosis).
Perceptually, her voice trails off/loses volume at the end of a phrase (symptom/functioning).
She complains of shortness of breath (SOB) while talking (patient complaint).

Any or all of these factors are reasons to focus on adduction exercises, breath support, control of airflow during speech, and phrasing.

Symptomatic voice therapy means treating the symptoms or problems associated with the problem. It is important to not only treat the diagnosis but to listen to the patient's vocal quality and watch for physical signs (e.g., posture, tension, strain, SOB). Training your ear is important in order to perceptually assess and address changes in vocal quality that may occur throughout the therapy process. It is important to maintain balance in the voice. For example, if you are treating a patient with a diagnosis of muscle tension dysphonia (MTD) and you are working on relaxation and increased airflow, you must use balanced therapy goals in order to avoid a breathy vocal quality. Maintaining this balance will often mean addressing multiple voice parameters at the same time.

The therapy tasks (production drills) in this chapter are organized into these sections:

- Respiration
- Phonation
- Resonance

This organization does not mean that these areas should be addressed separately in therapy. Most often you will be working on tasks from each section within one therapy session in order to achieve a balance of airflow, phonatory ease, and oral and nasal resonance. Even though one area may need more focus than another, keep all of these voice parameters in mind when choosing activities/targets.

*Clinical Note*: It is often best to work on breathing and airflow first, as this is the driving force of the voice.

Activities are designed for use within the therapy session. Your cueing and modeling are essential to facilitate and insure proper production of the desired target. Focus on a target to master, and probe the patient's ability to self-monitor her ability for correct production. It is helpful to have the patient rate productions within the therapy session and have her focus on how her voice sounds and/or feels when using target behaviors.

It is important to provide the patient with the "whys" of the exercises and tasks you are asking her to practice. For example, "We are working on cervical exercises to relax your neck and shoulder muscles. These muscles are often tense during breathing and voice use. We are working from the outside-in to relax your voice." This explanation will facilitate patient understanding and internalization of the concepts of voice production to allow for carryover and habituation into conversational speech. Daily practice of activities will aid the patient's ability to manipulate and monitor her voice.

Photocopy activities for home practice once the patient is able to hit the target with use of self-identification and monitoring. For some patients, it is helpful to audiotape or videotape them speaking to assist with self-identification of vocal quality.

The activities described in this chapter offer suggestions regarding the target, goal, and possible cueing strategies/instructions. However, you may also find other ways to use these stimuli in therapy.

## PHYSICAL EXERCISES

Physical exercises are often used before beginning voice therapy to reduce jaw/mandibular tension and cervical tension that may be a contributing factor in many hyperfunctional vocal conditions. These exercises also aid in promoting self-identification of tension and relaxation.

## Jaw Exercises

*Caution*:  Do not perform with patients who complain of temporomandibular joint (TMJ) pain.

Instructions to patient:

1.  Open your mouth wide.  Use slow, exaggerated movements.

2.  Chew as if you have taffy between your molars.  Use both up and down and circular movement of your lower jaw (rotary chewing).

## Palatal Exercise

Instructions to patient:

- Open your mouth as wide as you can.

- Raise your soft palate (the very back of your throat) as if you are going to yawn or are trying to fit a golf ball in the back of your throat.

- Hold for a count of 3 to 5 seconds.

## Shoulder Exercises (See illustrated instructions, page 96.)

## Cervical Exercises (See illustrated instructions, pages 97-100.)

## Adduction Exercises (See illustrated instructions, pages 101-102.)

# Shoulder Exercises

**Target**:  cervical relaxation

**Goal**:  reduction of upper body tension to promote extrinsic laryngeal relaxation

1. Shrug your shoulders, bringing them up toward your ears.

2. Roll your shoulders.  Bring both shoulders up toward your ears and then roll your shoulders backward and downward.

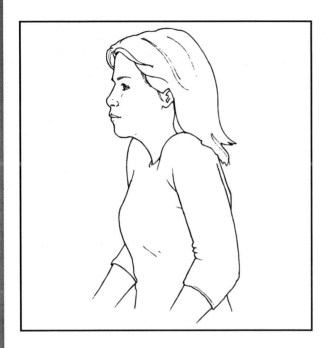

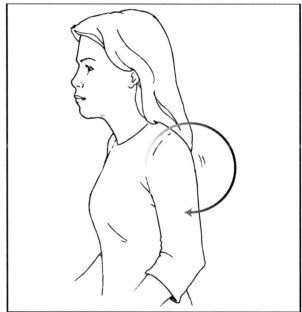

3. Keep your shoulders down and relaxed with your arms by your sides, and make exaggerated, slow swinging motions with your arms.

4. With your hands by your sides, bring your arms out straight to the side and up over your head.  Touch your palms together.

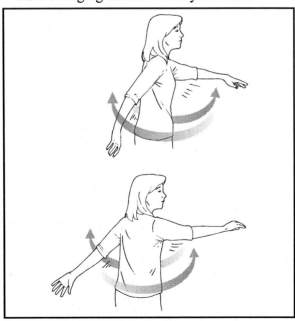

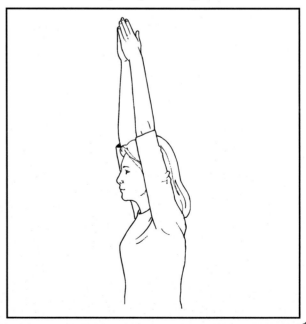

The Source for Voice Disorders
Adolescent & Adult

# Cervical Exercises

**Target**: extrinsic laryngeal tension

**Goal**: to stretch the extrinsic laryngeal muscles and promote relaxed laryngeal movement

## Head turn

1. Lie on your back on the floor or a hard surface.

2. Turn your head to the right, placing your right hand on your left cheekbone to add a slight resistance.

3. Stretch to look over your shoulder (do not stretch to the point of pain), keeping your left shoulder on the floor.

4. Repeat on the left, using your left hand against your right cheekbone and keeping your right shoulder on the floor.

5. Perform 10 times on each side.

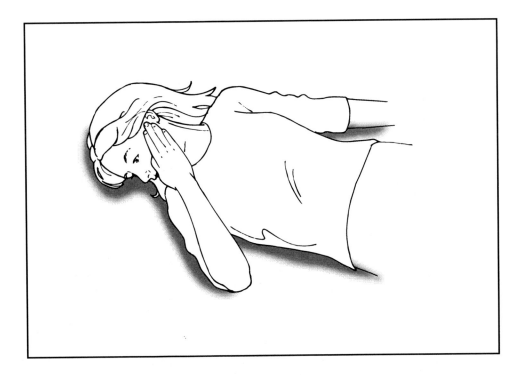

# Cervical Exercises

**Target**: extrinsic laryngeal tension

**Goal**: to stretch the extrinsic laryngeal muscles and promote relaxed laryngeal movement

## Head tilt

1. Lie on your back on the floor or a hard surface. Keep your shoulders on the floor.

2. Place your right hand over top of your head and slightly pull your head to touch your right ear to your right shoulder (tilting, not turning, your head). Bring your ear as close as you can to your shoulder without stretching to the point of pain. Tilt your neck, not your torso.

3. Repeat on the left side. Bring your left ear to your left shoulder, using your left hand over top of your head.

4. Perform 10 times on each side.

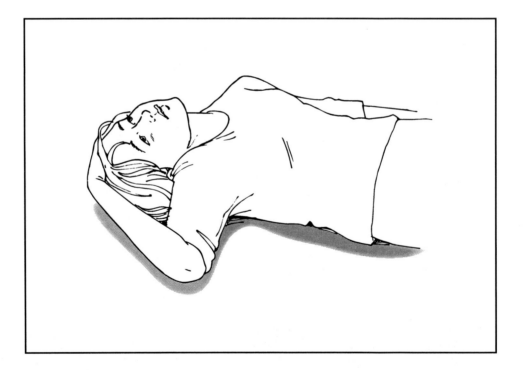

The Source for Voice Disorders
Adolescent & Adult

# Cervical Exercises

**Target**: extrinsic laryngeal tension

**Goal**: to stretch the extrinsic laryngeal muscles and promote relaxed laryngeal movement

## Lateral neck stretch

1. Stand upright and clasp your hands down low behind your back.

2. Turn your head to the right as far as you can and then slowly bring your chin up to look at the ceiling. Hold for a count of 3.

3. Bring your head to midline and repeat on the left. Turn your head to the left as far as you can and then slowly bring your chin up to look at the ceiling.

4. Repeat 10 times on each side.

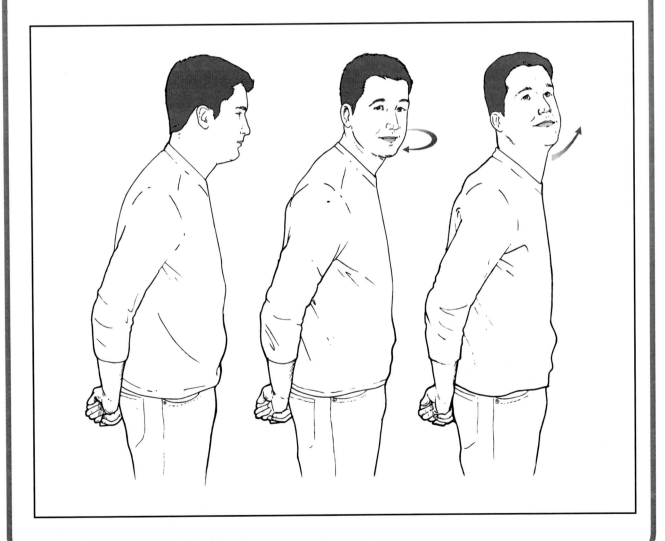

# Cervical Exercises

**Target**: extrinsic laryngeal tension

**Goal**: to stretch the extrinsic laryngeal muscles and promote relaxed laryngeal movement

## Chin to Chest

1. Stand upright and clasp your hands down low behind your back.

2. Keep your shoulders low and back and bring your chin to your chest.

3. Hold for a count of 5.

4. Repeat 10 times.

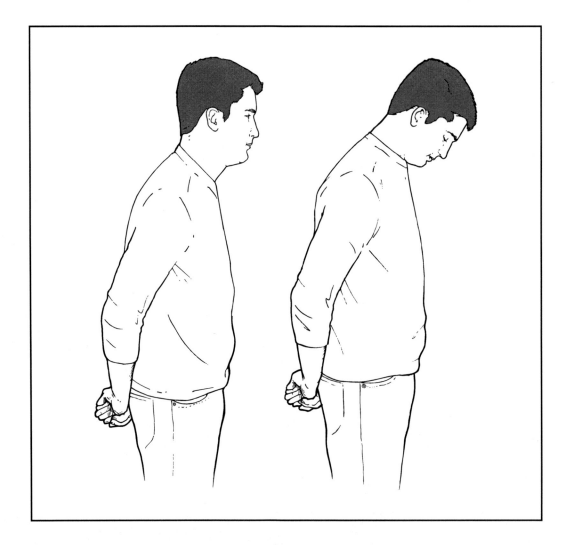

The Source for Voice Disorders
Adolescent & Adult

# Adduction Exercises

**Target**:        vocal fold (VF) adduction

**Goal**:        to improve medial glottal closure through the use of tension

**Background**:   Adduction exercises are most often used in hypofunctional voice disorders
(e.g., presbylarynx) and neurologic vocal conditions (e.g., vocal fold paralysis)
that result in reduced vocal fold adduction and/or reduced volume.

These exercises use pushing and/or pulling during phonation, resulting in increased
vocal fold closure and increased subglottic air pressure. Use this increased pressure
to produce a louder vocal tone.

*Clinical Note*: Take care not to strain the laryngeal or cervical muscles during these exercises. In
addition, do not do these exercises if the vocal folds are inflamed or a hyperfunctional pathology is
present, as in the case of vocal fold nodules or hemorrhage.

## Adduction Exercise 1

1. Sit in a straight back chair and clasp your hands in front of your chest.

2. Take a deep breath.

3. Try to pull your hands apart while holding a steady "ahhh" for 10 seconds.

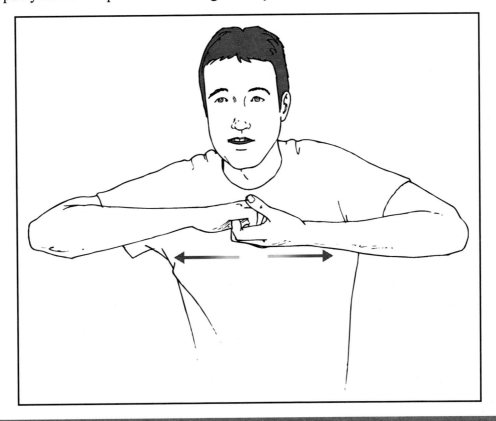

# Adduction Exercises

**Target**: vocal fold (VF) adduction

**Goal**: to improve medial glottal closure through the use of tension

## Adduction Exercise 2

1.  Sit in a straight back chair and place your hands under the seat of the chair.

2.  Take a deep breath.

3.  Pull up on the chair while holding a steady "ahhh" for 10 seconds.

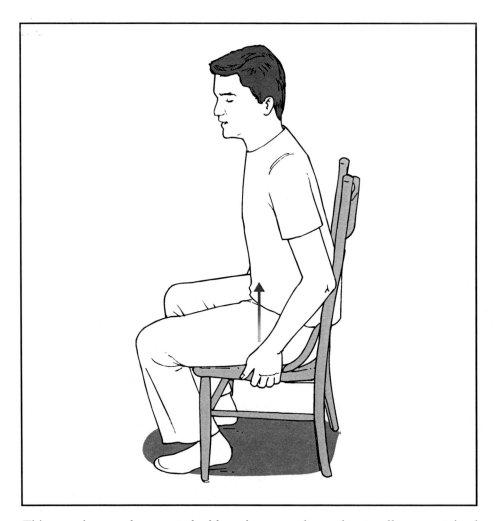

This exercise may be repeated with various vowel sounds as well as a sustained hum. Use increased volume on subsequent trials.

The Source for Voice Disorders
Adolescent & Adult

## OTHER USEFUL TECHNIQUES FOR VOCAL HYPOFUNCTION

a. Glottal attack/staccato production of vowels for rapid adduction

*Example*: Have the patient repeat "ee-ee-ee" using rapid, hard pulses of air through the vocal folds.

b. Use of loud phonation

*Example*: Have the patient produce words/sentences with increased volume.

c. Swallow and then phonate

*Example*: Instruct the patient to swallow, followed by an immediate "eeee" production.

d. Pitch glides and scales with vowel production

A glide is a slide through a series of pitches using continuous phonation.

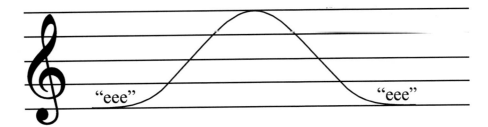

A pitch scale is a separate production of each note/pitch.

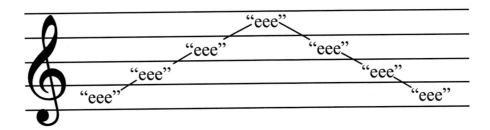

# Respiration Exercises

**Target:**      respiration/airflow

**Goal:**      to facilitate voice production

**Background:**      The technique of diaphragmatic breathing is the basis for easy voice production.

The diaphragm is the dome-shaped muscle that separates your lungs from your visceral organs (stomach, liver, intestines, kidneys). It is located at the bottom of your rib cage (See Figure 10, page 13, Chapter 1).

It is important to breathe using your diaphragm for many reasons:

- You are able to reach higher total lung volumes (more space) and inhale more air.
- It does not involve active chest or clavicular movement (doesn't involve external laryngeal muscles) and improves relaxation of the laryngeal posture.
- Support and control of air by the diaphragm reduces the need for laryngeal control of airflow.

## Diaphragmatic Breathing Practice

1. Lie on your back.
2. Place a book on your diaphragm.
3. Place one hand on the book and one hand on your chest.
4. Raise the book as you breathe IN without raising your chest.

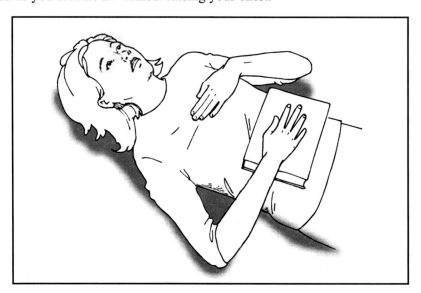

*Clinical Note*: Make sure that the patient is not contracting abdominal muscles to move the book but is using air to expand her lungs. Cue air exchange through the use of audible inhale/exhale (e.g., Have the patient purse her lips as she blows in and out to "hear" the movement of air).

The Source for Voice Disorders
Adolescent & Adult

# Respiration Exercises

**Target**: respiration/airflow

**Goal**: to learn airflow control techniques

**Background**: Once the patient has learned the technique of diaphragmatic breathing (page 104), it is important to learn control of airflow. The exhalation phase should be at least twice as long as the inhalation phase.

Inhale/exhale with a 1:2 ratio (count out loud to cue patient). Have the patient place his hand on the diaphragm for a tactile cue and/or have him use audible inhalation/ exhalation/pursed lips for an auditory cue.

## Inhalation/Exhalation Practice

**Cue**: "I will count out loud. I want you to inhale for 3 seconds and exhale for 6 seconds."

- Continue with the following intervals:    4 seconds/8 seconds
                                             5 seconds/10 seconds
                                             6 seconds/12 seconds

- Randomize trials above.

- Use a voiceless consonant to monitor exhalation (/s/).

- Use sustained phonation practice (/m/ or /a/).

# Respiration Exercises

**Target**: control of airflow during phonation

**Goal**: to use continuous and controlled airflow during controlled automatic speech tasks

## Airflow/Phonation Practice

**Cue**: "After a diaphragmatic breath, count from 1-20 out loud, taking a breath after every 5 numbers."

". . . 1-20 with a breath after every 4 numbers."

". . . 1-50 with a breath after every 10 numbers."

- Continue with other sets of multiples, asking the patient to control the coordination of breathing and voice use. Monitor vocal quality for evidence of strain or tension.

- If the patient is able to reach 10 numbers on one breath, have her count with voiceless onset/breathy consonants using controlled and continuous airflow. This task requires more airflow.

    Cue and model an aspirated initial consonant:

    "Count from 30-39 on one breath using a slightly extended, breathy /th/.

    "Count from 40-49 on one breath using a slightly extended, breathy /f/.

    "Count from 50-59 on one breath using a slightly extended, breathy /f/.

    "Count from 60-69 on one breath using a slightly extended, breathy /s/.

- Once the patient is able to perform these tasks in sets, have her "count from 30 to 80" taking a breath after every ten numbers. This task will aid in coordination of breathing during running speech.

The Source for Voice Disorders
Adolescent & Adult

# Respiration Exercises

**Target:** coordination of airflow

**Goal:** to reinforce the use of breath support and coordination of breathing during speaking

**Background:** Phrasing and meaning is usually determined by a speaker's use of pause. Often the breathing pattern is dictated by the text.

You can also practice pause and breathing patterns with nursery rhymes, poems, short songs, etc. For additional carryover, use materials such as newspapers and magazines where the "rhythm" is not established.

## Airflow Coordination Practice

**Cue:** "Read the 'Pledge of Allegiance' and take a breath at every slash (/) marked in the text. Make sure you are taking appropriate size breaths for the length of the utterance and remember to let air out as you talk."

**I pledge allegiance to the flag / of the United States of America / and to the republic for which it stands / one nation under God / indivisible with liberty / and justice for all.**

Now try it with a different breathing pattern:

**I pledge allegiance to the flag of the United States of America / and to the republic for which it stands / one nation under God / indivisible with liberty and justice for all.**

# Respiration Exercises

**Target:** coordination of airflow

**Goal:** to reinforce the use of breath support and coordination of breathing during speaking tasks of increasing length

**Background:** Have the patient read the following run-on sentence out loud and focus on the use of pauses to replenish airflow at semantically-appropriate breaks.

**Cue:** "The following sentence increases in length each time it is repeated. As the sentence gets longer, you will need to pause to take in air to complete the next phrase. Try to use natural pauses based on the meaning of the sentence."

## Sentence Length Phrasing Task

Excuse me.

Excuse me, miss.

Excuse me, miss, I need directions.

Excuse me, miss, I need directions to the store.

Excuse me, miss, I need directions to the store on Main Street.

Excuse me, miss, I need directions to the store on Main Street that sells toys.

Excuse me, miss, I need directions to the store on Main Street that sells toys for babies.

Excuse me, miss, I need directions to the store on Main Street that sells toys for babies and toddlers.

Excuse me, miss, I need directions to the store on Main Street that sells toys for babies and toddlers from a gift registry.

Excuse me, miss, I need directions to the store on Main Street that sells toys for babies and toddlers from a gift registry for expectant mothers.

Excuse me, miss, I need directions to the store on Main Street that sells toys for babies and toddlers from a gift registry for expectant mothers who need essentials.

Excuse me, miss, I need directions to the store on Main Street that sells toys for babies and toddlers from a gift registry for expectant mothers who need essentials and are hoping for a shower.

Excuse me, miss, I need directions to the store on Main Street that sells toys for babies and toddlers from a gift registry for expectant mothers who need essentials and are hoping for a shower to receive gifts.

Excuse me, miss, I need directions to the store on Main Street that sells toys for babies and toddlers from a gift registry for expectant mothers who need essentials and are hoping for a shower to receive gifts from families and friends.

Excuse me, miss, I need directions to the store on Main Street that sells toys for babies and toddlers from a gift registry for expectant mothers who need essentials and are hoping for a shower to receive gifts from families and friends because having a baby is very expensive.

Excuse me, miss, I need directions to the store on Main Street that sells toys for babies and toddlers from a gift registry for expectant mothers who need essentials and are hoping for a shower to receive gifts from families and friends because having a baby is very expensive these days.

The Source for Voice Disorders
Adolescent & Adult

# Respiration Exercises

**Target:**  airflow (to be used with patients who exhibit glottal attack or hard/tense onset of phonation)

**Goal:**  to start airflow prior to voicing in order to reduce tension associated with voice production

**Background:**  Have the patient initiate voice on an aspirated /h/ to start airflow prior to phonation. Cue for continuous airflow throughout word production. The voice should not sound breathy or whispered.

Once the patient is able to start airflow on an extended /h/, have him shorten the word to a normal rate but continue to "think air on the H."

**Cue:**  "Hold the /h/ sound slightly longer than normal to get your air started and then say the word. Continue to exhale and let the air out during the word. Continue the air from the H into the vowel that follows."

## H Words—Single Syllables
### Example:  "hhhhair"

| | | | |
|---|---|---|---|
| hail | hawk | herd | hoist |
| hair | haze | hide | hold |
| half | head | high | hole |
| hall | heal | hill | home |
| halt | health | hike | hood |
| ham | heart | him | hoof |
| hand | hearth | hind | hoop |
| Hank | heave | hint | hoot |
| hard | heed | hip | hop |
| harm | height | hit | hope |
| harsh | help | hitch | horn |
| hash | hem | hive | horse |
| haste | hen | hoax | how |
| hate | her | hoe | hump |
| haul | Herb | hog | hush |

# Respiration Exercises

**Target:** airflow (to be used with patients who exhibit glottal attack or hard/tense onset of phonation)

**Goal:** to start airflow prior to voicing in order to reduce tension associated with voice production

**Background:** Have the patient practice with extended /h/ until airflow is promoted, and then shorten the word to a normal rate of production but continue to "think H."

---

**Cue:** "These words are longer so be sure to let air out through both syllables."

## H Words—2 Syllables
Example: "hhhhockey"

| | | | |
|---|---|---|---|
| habit | hateful | heartless | hollow |
| hairbrush | haven | helmet | holly |
| halfway | having | hermit | holster |
| hammock | Hawthorne | hero | homesick |
| hamstring | hazard | hiding | homespun |
| handy | hazing | highway | honey |
| happy | headache | himself | hopeful |
| harness | heading | hippo | hormone |
| hasten | headstone | hockey | hula |
| hatchet | healthy | holler | hygiene |

# Respiration Exercises

**Target:**   airflow (to be used with patients who exhibit glottal attack or hard/tense onset of phonation)

**Goal:**   to obtain continuous airflow throughout sentences of increasing length

**Background:**   Use modeling to promote correct production.

> Incorrect: "Honk the horn." (pause in air between words)
> Correct: "Honk-the-horn" (continuous airflow)

---

**Cue:**   "Let's work on phrases and sentences. Continue to let air out through the whole phrase without stopping your air between words."

## H Phrases and Sentences

| | |
|---|---|
| Hit his head | He hated hurricanes. |
| Honk the horn. | Hope for hot ham hash. |
| Hitchhike home. | Hobby horses hop high. |
| Hum a harmony. | Honeymoon in Houston |
| Hearths have heat. | Heartthrob in Hollywood |
| Hail hit the house. | Henry hid the horseradish. |
| Help Hillary home. | Hal hula-hoops to Hawaii. |
| Held her head high | Hank's home is on the hill. |
| Helmets hide heads. | Hamburgers and hot chocolate |
| Hear his hypothesis. | Her hockey skate hurt her heel. |
| Harriet held the hen. | Horrible hair for Homecoming |
| Horses have hooves. | He hates honeybees and hornets. |
| Hold the handlebars. | He was hesitant to hypnotize her. |
| Hot, humid Honduras | Herman had horrible handwriting. |
| Hanna hates this hairbrush. | Heather is a homemaker in New Hampshire. |

**Target**: airflow (to be used with patients who exhibit glottal attack or hard/tense onset of phonation)

**Goal**: to obtain continuous airflow throughout sentences of increasing length

**Cue**: "The following sentences contain multiple F sounds. Practice using continuous airflow throughout each sentence. Use slightly extended /f/ productions."

## F Phrases and Sentences

Fred fishes for flounder.

Florists sell fresh flowers.

Her fingers dialed the phone.

Fortune tellers tell the future.

The family enjoyed the feast.

Pharmacists fill prescriptions.

Four golf balls fell in the ferns.

The fern leaf blew off the cliff.

The fawn frolicked in the forest.

Felix the feline feasted on a fish.

Family photographs fill the frames.

Five first graders started a food fight.

Farmers put fences around their fields.

The chef cut the fish filet with a knife.

The fig filling made a fantastic dessert.

I found a fancy ruffled dress for the festival.

The firefighter fought the fire from the roof.

The fiberglass furnace filter was filled with fuzz.

For breakfast, fresh coffee and waffles fill me up fast.

Jeff found the finest office furniture on the sales floor.

Fashionable fabrics were featured in the fashion show.

When you cough, cover your mouth with a handkerchief.

Upon finding the fortune in the safe, the sheriff handcuffed the thief.

Phyllis forgot about her fourth physics assignment on the forces of flight.

The forty-year-old female filed her fingernails on the front porch of the farmhouse.

# Respiration Exercises

**Target:**  airflow (to be used with patients who exhibit glottal attack or hard/tense onset of phonation)

**Goal:**  to obtain continuous airflow throughout sentences of increasing length

**Cue:**  "The following sentences contain multiple S sounds.  Practice using continuous airflow throughout each sentence.  Use slightly extended /s/ productions."

## S Phrases and Sentences

Sweet juice sells fast.

Saddles rest on horses.

Soft sounds soothe the class.

Sell some socks and sunglasses.

Surfers ride the surf into the sand.

Sing the first verse of the silly song.

Sara signaled for the shoe salesperson.

Sports cars swerve when going too fast.

Search for the satin slippers in the store.

Sam scouted the produce section for celery.

Susan was so anxious waiting to sing on stage.

Sixteen silk suits were sold during the spring sale.

Serious servants separate soiled linens from the rest.

Congress passed the bill to save the southern sea seals.

Scrap silverware satisfies scavengers who seek small stuff.

Scott secretly signed his sloppy signature on the assignment.

Baseball, basketballs, and bicycles were spread out on the grass.

The lighthouse beam shined brilliantly across the sea to warn cautious sailors.

Sue slurped strawberry shakes at the skating rink every Sunday from six until seven.

While sitting helpless in the safe, the boss of the business was saved by the city police.

# Phonation Exercises

**Target**: continuous voicing

**Goal**: to elicit continuous vibration/phonation

**Background**: The following words only contain voiced consonants to promote continuous vibration of the vocal folds.  Listen for breaks in phonation.

---

**Cue**: "The following words require your vocal folds to vibrate without any breaks.  Say the following words and continue easy phonation."

## Continuous Voiced Words

| | | | |
|---|---|---|---|
| bored | eardrum | lazy | these |
| Bradley | earrings | living | those |
| breezy | endearing | Louisiana | Virginia |
| daisy | games | margin | vision |
| David | gaze | muzzle | void |
| dazed | geranium | olives | zebra |
| diary | gleaming | raisin | Zelda |
| diving board | grades | remember | zig-zag |
| driving | Irving | roses | zoology |

# Phonation Exercises

**Target:**    continuous voicing

**Goal:**    to maintain vibration using voiced continuants

**Background:**    The following phrases and sentences contain multiple voiced continuants (/v/ and /z/) to promote vocal fold vibration.

---

**Cue:**    "The following phrases and sentences contain multiple /v/ and /z/ consonant sounds. Focus on maintaining the vibration of your voice."

| V Phrases/Sentences | Z Phrases/Sentences |
|---|---|
| Very valuable | Zebras at the zoo |
| Vicki's violets | His knees are bruised. |
| Beverly and Victor | Knows the ZIP code |
| Vacation in November | Zoe has a xylophone. |
| Lives in Vienna | Liz plays jazz. |
| A villa in the valley | Zack is a zoologist. |
| Yvonne drives a Volvo. | Zip up his zipper. |
| Vinnie believes in vampires. | These are lazy days. |

# Phonation Exercises

**Target:** voiceless-voiced transitions

**Goals:** to increase awareness of vocal fold vibration
to improve transition from a voiceless consonant to a voiced vowel sound

**Background:** A patient will often have difficulty "getting her voice started" after a voiceless consonant. The following tasks will aid in patient self-monitoring and awareness of the onset of the voice.

**Task 1:** Have the patient produce a sustained phoneme in isolation to contrast voiceless with voiced productions.

**Cue:** "Say and hold a /s/ sound (model "ssss"). Now say and hold a /z/ sound (model "zzzz"). Feel the difference on the /z/ when your vocal folds vibrate versus a /s/, which is mostly air."

**Task 2:** Have the patient read the following list of words to contrast "voiced" vs. "voiceless" productions.

**Cue:** "Read these words in pairs and focus on increased airflow on the second word without pushing your voice on the vowel sound."

## Voiced and Voiceless Minimal Pairs

| Voiced | Voiceless | Voiced | Voiceless |
|--------|-----------|--------|-----------|
| vat | fat | zip | sip |
| veal | feel | zing | sing |
| vine | fine | zoo | Sue |
| van | fan | zeal | seal |
| vase | face | Zeke | seek |
| vault | fault | Zack | sack |
| vend | fend | zinc | sink |
| veil | fail | zit | sit |
| vast | fast | zap | sat |
| | | zoot | suit |

# Phonation Exercises

**Target:** voiceless-voiced transitions

**Goals:** to increase awareness of vocal fold vibration
to improve transition from a voiceless consonant to a voiced vowel sound

**Background:** A patient will often have difficulty "getting his voice started" after a voiceless consonant. The following tasks will aid in patient self-monitoring and awareness of the onset of the voice.

**Cue:** "Read these words in pairs and focus on the easy phonation on the first word without pushing your voice on the vowel sound."

## Voiceless and Voiced Minimal Pairs

| Voiceless | Voiced | Voiceless | Voiced |
|-----------|--------|-----------|--------|
| tame | dame | came | game |
| tomb | doom | Kate | gate |
| tot | dot | cut | gut |
| tuck | duck | come | gum |
| ton | done | kilt | guilt |
| team | deem | kill | gill |
| pat | bat | call | gall |
| pump | bump | cheap | jeep |
| pass | bass | chive | jive |
| punch | bunch | choke | joke |
| push | bush | chunk | junk |
| Pete | beat | chug | jug |
| puck | buck | chill | Jill |
| pack | back | chest | jest |
| pounce | bounce | chin | gin |
| pit | bit | | |

# Phonation Exercises

**Target:** voiceless-voiced transitions

**Goal:** to encourage the easy transitions from voiceless consonants to voiced vowels

**Background:** The following words contain only voiceless consonants (no vocal fold vibration). Listen for pitch or aphonic breaks going into the vowels and/or vocal strain.

**Cue:** "The following words contain consonant sounds that do not require vocal fold vibration. Use airflow from the consonants to produce easy vowel sounds."

## Voiceless Consonant Words

| | |
|---|---|
| ashes | poppy |
| caps | potty |
| Cathy | puffy |
| faith | push |
| fast | sachet |
| fifty-two | sassy |
| fishy | Scottish |
| happy | shaft |
| Hawaii | soup |
| Heath | spaceship |
| hip-hop | teeth |
| hope | thick |
| hotel | thief |
| kitty cat | thought |
| pasta | ticket |
| Patty | tick-tock |
| peace | whip |
| physics | whiskey |
| pity | without |

# Phonation Exercises

**Target:**     easy onset/reduction of glottal attack

**Goal:**     to produce easy onset of words starting with vowels in order to reduce tension

**Background:** Patients exhibiting hyperfunctional voice disorders often have difficulty with vowel-initial words because all vowels are "voiced" and certain vowels are tense (vs. lax) in production (short vowels are often more difficult than long vowels).

---

**Task 1:** Have the patient say the following word pairs in order to encourage airflow/reduce glottal attack when initiating the voice on a vowel sound.

> **Cue:** "Now that you have learned to start your voice using air, I want you to do that with sounds that are not breathy. All of the following words start with vowels. Practice using an 'H' first and then taking the 'H' away, but still use air to get your voice started."
>
> *Example:*   heat/eat
> (The vowel should sound the same in both words without hard attack/onset on the second word.)

**Task 2:** Have the patient say just the vowel onset words as you listen for glottal attack and cue for airflow.

> **Cue:** "Now say just the words that begin with vowels, but still let air out first to start your voice easy."

## Easy Onset Practice

| | |
|---|---|
| hail • ale | heel • eel |
| hair • air | high • I |
| hall • all | hike • Ike |
| ham • am | hill • ill |
| harm • arm | his • is |
| has • as | hit • it |
| hear • ear | hive • I've |
| heat • eat | how • ow |

# Phonation Exercises

**Target**:  easy onset of vowels—connected phonation

**Goal**:  to maintain production of easy onset/reduce glottal attack of vowels throughout sentence production

**Note**:  This exercise should follow easy onset practice at the word level.

---

**Cue**:  "The following phrases and sentences contain multiple words that start with vowels.  Use the same techniques of easy onset, airflow, and relaxed voicing throughout the sentence.  Do not start and stop your voice."  (Voice quality should not sound staccato.)

## Vowel Onset Phrases/Sentences

Open up.

in and out

all around

over and out

artist's easel

another option

eager adolescents

Open an envelope.

ingenious ideas

Einstein's inventions

all of your efforts

extremely egotistical

impossible expectation

Another option always exists.

Ellen is always around at Easter.

Our Uncle Alan is always angry.

It is impossible to understand arithmetic.

Eric's umbrella is under the overhang.

Astronauts are unbelievably ambitious.

Everyone asks if Amy is my aunt.

I'll have already eaten enough oatmeal.

Emma is an unusually artistic adolescent.

If you enter early, attendants are available in the aisles.

Actors arrive at the awards in expensive attire.

Accountants are always extremely accurate.

Ethan and Ivana are always at the opera.

Olivia was embarrassed by all of Arthur's attention.

It was an eye-opening experience for Allison.

It is an effort to understand Uncle Edward's accent.

Otto's used automobiles are usually under eight thousand dollars.

The Source for Voice Disorders
Adolescent & Adult

# Phonation Exercises

**Target:**   easy onset of vowels—paragraph level

**Goal:**   to maintain production of easy onset/reduce glottal attack of vowels throughout a connected speech task (also monitor coordination of breath support and phrasing)

**Background:**   This exercise should follow easy onset practice at the phrase and sentence level.

**Cue:**   "The following paragraph contains mostly words that start with vowel sounds. Use the same techniques of easy onsets and relaxed voicing that you did during the vowel sentence reading tasks, but remember to replenish your breath support to allow for running speech."

## Vowel Intense Paragraph

Emma Oliver is approximately eleven years old. As many other adolescent girls, Emma is overly concerned about her appearance. Every afternoon, Emma asks to be excused to use the ladies' room to insure that everything is "just so." It is unacceptable not to be one of the "in crowd" and being attractive assures your inclusion. Even at the early age of eleven, a girl allows herself to be influenced by others. Emma's mother always asks her "Why is it so important to be like everyone else?" "It just is! You wouldn't understand because you are old," answers Emma. At age eleven, anyone over thirty is old.

# Phonation Exercises

**Target**: intonation

**Goals**: to promote self-monitoring of rising vs. falling intonation
to maintain pitch stability on sentence endings (avoid glottal fry)

**Background**: In the English language a drop in pitch signifies the end of a phrase or sentence. Have the patient monitor her voice so it doesn't drop too low at the end.

**Cue**: "Say these two sentences as a pair, the first as a question and the second as a statement. Be careful not to drop your pitch too low on the endings."

## Intonation Practice—Sentences

You want to go to the park?

You want to go to the park.


I have to pay my bills on Wednesday?

I have to pay my bills on Wednesday.


His mother's name is Susan?

His mother's name is Susan.


The visiting team won the game?

The visiting team won the game.


Tomorrow we will have the party?

Tomorrow we will have the party.


Audrey cut her hair short?

Audrey cut her hair short.


There is no more room in this cabinet?

There is no more room in this cabinet.


It has been six months since we last spoke?

It has been six months since we last spoke.


Someone is knocking at the door?

Someone is knocking at the door.


Your prom dress is lavender?

Your prom dress is lavender.


It is too late to call her at home?

It is too late to call her at home.


Kimberly's cat has had kittens?

Kimberly's cat has had kittens.

# Phonation Exercises

**Target:**      pitch vs. volume/inflection

**Goals:**      to use intonation to emphasize a word within a running sentence
to improve use of stress (without volume or "push") and vocal variability

**Background:**   The following sentences are organized in sets. Have the patient emphasize the word that is in **bold**.

*Clinical Note:* If the patient has difficulty with emphasis on a single word, use the questions on the next page to elicit the desired intonational pattern.

---

**Cue:**    "Say the following sentence sets. Emphasize the word that is in bold letters. Use **pitch** inflection to stress that word—not **volume**."

## Intonation Practice—Words

**My** kitten's name is Casey.

My **kitten's** name is Casey.

My kitten's name is **Casey**.


**Jack** goes to college in Pittsburgh.

Jack goes to **college** in Pittsburgh.

Jack goes to college in **Pittsburgh**.


**I** have to work at 8 a.m. on Thursday.

I have to **work** at 8 a.m. on Thursday.

I have to work at **8 a.m.** on Thursday.

I have to work at 8 a.m. on **Thursday**.


**Phillip's** hobby is antique car repair.

Phillip's **hobby** is antique car repair.

Phillip's hobby is antique **car** repair.

Phillip's hobby is antique car **repair**.


I would like a **silver** bracelet for graduation.

I would like a silver **bracelet** for graduation.

I would like a silver bracelet for **graduation**.


**Eric** painted his bedroom blue.

Eric **painted** his bedroom blue

Eric painted **his** bedroom blue.

Eric painted his **bedroom** blue.

Eric painted his bedroom **blue**.

# Phonation Exercises

**Target**:          pitch vs. volume/inflection

**Goals**:          to use intonation to emphasize a word within a running sentence
to improve use of stress (without volume or "push") and vocal variability

**Background**:   Present the questions in the right column below to elicit the desired response from the patient (left column). Give the patient page 123 to read.

---

**Cue**:      "Say the following sentence sets. Emphasize the word that is in bold letters. Use **pitch** inflection to stress that word—not **volume**."

## Intonation Practice—Words

| *Patient* | *Clinician* |
|---|---|
| **My** kitten's name is Casey. | Is **his** kitten's name Casey? |
| My **kitten's** name is Casey. | Is your **dog's** name Casey? |
| My kitten's name is **Casey**. | Is your kitten's name **Fluffy**? |
| | |
| **Jack** goes to college in Pittsburgh. | Does **Susan** go to college in Pittsburgh? |
| Jack goes to **college** in Pittsburgh. | Does Jack go to **camp** in Pittsburgh? |
| Jack goes to college in **Pittsburgh**. | Does Jack go to college in **Virginia**? |
| | |
| **I** have to work at 8 a.m. on Thursday. | Does your **wife** have to work at 8 a.m. on Thursday? |
| I have to **work** at 8 a.m. on Thursday. | Do you have to **swim** at 8 a.m. on Thursday? |
| I have to work at **8 a.m.** on Thursday. | Do you have to work at **9 a.m.** on Thursday? |
| I have to work at 8 a.m. on **Thursday**. | Do you have to work at 8 a.m. on **Tuesday**? |
| | |
| **Phillip's** hobby is antique car repair. | Is **John's** hobby antique car repair? |
| Phillip's **hobby** is antique car repair. | Is Phillip's **occupation** antique car repair? |
| Phillip's hobby is antique **car** repair. | Is Phillip's hobby antique **train** repair? |
| Phillip's hobby is antique car **repair**. | Is Phillip's hobby antique car **sales**? |
| | |
| I would like a **silver** bracelet for graduation. | Would you like a **gold** bracelet for graduation? |
| I would like a silver **bracelet** for graduation. | Would you like a silver **ring** for graduation? |
| I would like a silver bracelet for **graduation**. | Would you like a silver bracelet for your **birthday**? |
| | |
| **Eric** painted his bedroom blue. | Did **Sam** paint his bedroom blue? |
| Eric **painted** his bedroom blue | Did Eric **wallpaper** his bedroom blue? |
| Eric painted **his** bedroom blue. | Did Eric paint **your** bedroom blue? |
| Eric painted his **bedroom** blue. | Did Eric paint his **bathroom** blue? |
| Eric painted his bedroom **blue**. | Did Eric paint his bedroom **green**? |

# Resonance Exercises

**Target:**  resonance

**Goals:**  to establish a more forward voice focus and improve vibratory sensations in the face (and alveolar ridge)

to reduce laryngeal focus (the vocal folds are in an easy, adducted position—not pressed or forced hyperadduction)

**Background:**  Have the patient place his fingers on each side of his nose on the facial bones and produce a hum (/m/) to get tactile feedback and focus vibration. The patient may need to adjust his pitch to obtain maximal vibration.

**Cue:**  "I want you to hum and feel the vibration in your face. Notice how you are not pushing from your larynx but achieving a resonant, clear vocal tone."

## Tactile Vibration

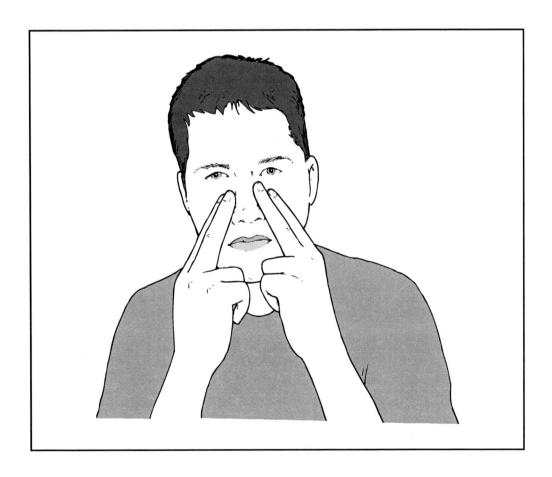

# Resonance Exercises

**Target**:        nasal vs. oral resonance

**Goals**:        to promote both nasal and oral resonance
to reduce laryngeal focus

**Background**:  Once the patient is able to hum and maintain forward focus, practice adding a vowel.

---

**Cue**:  "Say the following syllables. Start with a hum to focus your voice and produce the vowel with an open throat. Think about opening the space in the back of your throat to produce the vowel."

> *Examples*:    mmmmaaaa
> mmmmaaay
> mmmmeeeee
> mmmmoooo

## M — Single Syllables

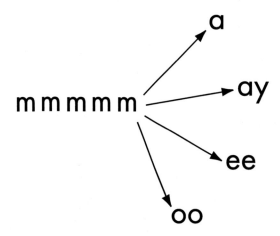

The Source for Voice Disorders
Adolescent & Adult
Copyright © 2004 LinguiSystems, Inc.

# Resonance Exercises

**Target**: resonance/reduce laryngeal focus

**Goals**: to promote the use of resonant voicing
to refocus vibration away from the larynx during phonation

**Cue**: "When you hum, your larynx is in a relaxed state. Start all of the following words on a hum and carry it through the word without dropping your voice into your throat."

## M — one-syllable words
*Example*: mmmmash

| | | |
|---|---|---|
| mad | meek | monk |
| made | melt | month |
| mail | merge | mood |
| main | mess | moon |
| make | met | moose |
| mall | mild | mop |
| malt | mile | more |
| man | milk | moss |
| map | mind | most |
| mare | mine | moth |
| mark | mink | mound |
| mash | mint | mourn |
| mask | mist | mouse |
| mass | mix | mouth |
| match | mob | move |
| may | mode | munch |
| meal | mold | mush |
| mean | mole | must |
| meat | mom | my |

# Resonance Exercises

**Target**: resonance/reduce laryngeal focus

**Goals**: to promote the use of resonant voicing
to refocus vibration away from the larynx during phonation

**Cue**: "Continue using your forward, resonant voice on these longer words.  Start your voice on a hum if you need to establish a higher vibration."

## M — two-syllable words
*Example*: mmmmother

| | | |
|---|---|---|
| machine | member | mohawk |
| magic | memo | moldy |
| maiden | menace | molten |
| mailbag | merger | monarch |
| major | merit | money |
| mango | messy | monkey |
| manmade | metric | monster |
| maple | middle | moody |
| market | mighty | moonbeam |
| marshall | million | morning |
| mascot | mindless | mouthpiece |
| master | minute | movie |
| matchbox | misread | mower |
| measure | mitten | muscle |
| meatloaf | mixer | music |
| melon | mobile | musty |
| melted | model | myself |

The Source for Voice Disorders
Adolescent & Adult
Copyright © 2004 LinguiSystems, Inc.

# Resonance Exercises

**Target:** resonance/reduce laryngeal focus

**Goal:** to maintain use of resonance and reduce laryngeal focus during sentence production

**Cue:** "Let's try phrases and sentences using a resonant voice. Remember to keep the vibration in your oral and nasal cavities—away from your throat."

## M Phrases & Sentences

My money

Many moons

Meet my mom.

My Mother Mary

March on Main Street.

Make me a maple malt.

Meet the men at the mine.

Muddy mowers make a mess.

Musicians' mouthpieces make music.

Magnify the marble with a microscope.

Military messengers sent the memos to me.

Mountain climbers are mystified by monumental peaks.

## Nasal Intense Sentences

My name is Nina.

Meet me at noon.

No more nickels and dimes.

Mike needs a hammer and nails.

Mom is mopping the sunroom.

My morning alarm makes music.

Mona makes mango jam in the summer.

Melanie may not need the microphone.

Kim and Mimi make money knitting mittens.

Matthew and Samantha might not come on Monday night.

# Oral Resonance Exercises

**Targets:** self-identification
reinforcement of oral resonance using vowel sounds

**Goals:** to facilitate the use of a relaxed oropharyngeal posture to improve oral resonance
to practice an "open-mouth" posture during vowel production

**Cue:** "The following words and short phrases contain vowels that are open or more relaxed. Focus on opening the back of your throat to produce these vowels. Relax the back of your tongue to increase the space in the back of your mouth." (Model "over-exaggerated" vowel production.)

## Open Vowels

### Words

| | | | |
|---|---|---|---|
| phone | spoon | bomb | roam |
| slow | sleuth | taught | woven |
| comb | shoe | boss | loft |
| stove | loose | blue | trauma |
| show | soon | suit | lost |
| loan | truth | choose | slot |
| toe | chose | loot | smog |
| hose | post | food | hot |
| soft | roll | zoom | moss |
| brought | home | smooth | dot |
| shot | boat | booth | whose |
| stop | smoke | moose | mood |
| pot | mold | snow | hoop |
| blot | poem | blow | doom |
| pod | drop | rope | goose |
| plot | Tom | load | loop |
| common | rod | coat | tomb |
| loom | dog | foam | Zeus |
| stoop | spot | cough | deuce |

### Phrases

blue suit
whose loot
soup spoon
common law
lost shoe
zoom zoom
tall Tom
all talk
too soon
tow rope
new boat
bomb squad
hot stove
go home
slow poke
cold snow
pawn shop
long rod
loose coat

The Source for Voice Disorders
Adolescent & Adult
Copyright © 2004 LinguiSystems, Inc.

# Oral Resonance Exercises

**Targets:**    reduction of laryngeal tension during the production of tense vowel sounds
use of increased oral resonance to reduce laryngeal tension

**Goals:**    to self identify tension and use a more relaxed laryngeal posture during the
production of tense vowels
to improve oral resonance and increase easy airflow on the production of tense vowels

**Background:**    Contrast this task with open vowels (page 130).

**Cue:**    "The following words contain vowels that are tighter or more tense in their production.
Continue to use an open throat as you say these words and phrases."

## Tense Vowels

| Words | | Phrases | |
|---|---|---|---|
| **/ae/** | **/ee/** | **/ae/** | **/ee/** |
| mast | sneeze | tax man | clean sweep |
| sat | seat | bad rash | team meet |
| bad | treat | sat back | lean meat |
| dash | seize | fat cat | eat wheat |
| sap | stream | fast track | please read |
| fat | eat | black saddle | sweet treat |
| track | please | dad's lap | steam heat |
| bat | release | tack back | tree leaf |
| practice | clean | vast land | keep neat |
| vat | piece | | |
| vast | speech | | |
| past | beam | | |
| rat | beak | | |
| rash | sleeve | | |
| cash | spree | | |
| fact | wheeze | | |
| slap | police | | |
| saddle | sweet | | |
| catch | steam | | |
| bash | seam | | |
| dad | weep | | |
| stash | feet | | |
| fast | week | | |
| sack | tree | | |
| smack | beet | | |
| lap | team | | |
| battle | easel | | |

## ADDITIONAL ORAL RESONANCE TECHNIQUES

The following are additional techniques to use with the patient to improve oral resonance:

- Yawn-sigh technique (page 92)
- Open-mouthed production of sustained "open vowels" (/a, ou, oo/)
- Practice of trills—this practice will focus vibration away from the larynx

    tongue trills

    lip trills

- Over-exaggeration of oral movements during practice
- Yodeling

## CARRYOVER

Once the patient has completed a therapy program designed to improve use of optimal airflow (respiration), voicing (phonation), and resonance techniques, it is imperative that the newly established vocal quality is used in everyday speaking. The following are some ideas for use in carryover:

- conversation
- role playing
- dialogue reading
- speaking in noise
- telephone use

# Recommendations for Teachers

### Reduce Background Noise

- Close windows and doors.
- Turn off unnecessary equipment (e.g., computers, overhead projectors).
- Make use of room decorations that absorb extraneous sound (e.g., curtains, rugs, student projects, wall hangings).
- Give students a specific time to gather belongings at the beginning of class in order to decrease background noise (e.g., rustling papers, backpack zippers).

### Classroom Modifications

- Use marker boards to reduce the effects of chalk dust (e.g., allergies, dryness).
- Run a classroom humidifier (if allowed).
- Position student seating around your primary speaking position (circular seating vs. rows).
- Use classroom amplification.

### Teaching Modifications

- Incorporate quiet reading, student projects, and question/answer sessions into your teaching style to build in "vocal rest time."
- Maintain good hydration while speaking.
- Don't talk through a cold or laryngitis. Use these days as "non-lecture" days.
- Use visual outlines and handouts to decrease verbal repetition of concepts/definitions.
- Use nonverbal cues to gain attention (e.g, ring a bell, turn lights off and on).
- Modify your teaching schedule. Break up lecture periods with labs and "hands on" electives for periods of vocal rest.

## References

Mattiske, J., Oates, J., & Greenwood, K. (1998). Vocal problems among teachers: A review of prevalence, causes, prevention, and treatment. *Journal of Voice, 12*, 489-499.

Martin, S. & Darley, L. (1996). *The teaching voice.* San Diego, CA: Singular Publishing.

McCabe, D. & Titze, I. (2002). Chant therapy for treating vocal fatigue among public school teachers: A preliminary study. *American Journal of Speech-Language Pathology, 11*, 4.

National Center for Voice & Speech (2003). *www.voiceacademy.org*

Roy, N., Weinrich, B., Gray, S., Tanner, K., Toledo, S., Dove, H., Corbin-Lewis, K., & Stemple, J. (2002). Voice amplification versus vocal hygiene instruction for teachers with voice disorders: A treatment outcomes study. *Journal of Speech, Language, and Hearing Research, 45*, 4.

# Terminology for the Singing Voice (Singer's Jargon)

The following is a brief list of terms used by vocalists.

**placement**:      use of forward focus to feel the vibrations of the facial bones

**chest register**:      singing in the lower range with heavy tones for louder singing

**head register**:      light tones used in soft or high singing

**full voice**:      singing at maximum volume and capacity

**marking**:      rehearsal singing; without use of full voice

**mezza voice**:      singing with half-voice

**legato**:      smooth and connected

**staccato**:      each note separated

**vibrato**:      rapidly fluctuating or pulsating quality (regular oscillation between two notes)

**falsetto**:      adjustment in technique to obtain the highest notes of the male voice

**alto**:      the lowest-pitched female singing voice

**bass**:      the lowest-pitched male singing voice

**baritone**:      range slightly higher than a bass

**soprano**:      the highest-pitched female singing voice

**mezzo soprano**:      slightly lower than a soprano

**tenor**:      the highest-pitched male singing voice

Adapted from *The Visible Voice*, Volume 1, No. 4, October 1992.

# Care of the Singing Voice

- It is important that you drink a minimum of 64 oz. of water a day. Your urine should be clear if you are adequately hydrated. Steam inhalers are a convenient way to add additional moisture directly to your vocal tract.

- Limit your intake of caffeine and alcohol. They dehydrate the tissues in your body. You need to drink an equal size glass of water for every caffeinated or alcoholic beverage you drink to counteract the drying effects (in addition to your 8-10 glasses).

- Some medications can be drying to the vocal fold tissue and mucosa. Singing on dehydrated vocal fold tissue can lead to increased effort for singing and can put you at risk for a vocal fold injury. Antihistamines (taken for colds, sinus and allergy symptoms) are the best examples of this. Use these medications only with a lot of water (80+ oz.) and sparingly.

- Singers should avoid aspirin products at all times. This includes any anti-inflammatory drugs, such as Aleve, Motrin, or Advil. These agents thin the blood and predispose one to sustain a vocal fold hemorrhage, particularly if coupled with excessive voice use or with improper voice use. Tylenol (acetaminophen) is acceptable.

- Frequent throat clearing and coughing are abusive to the vocal folds and can injure the vocal fold tissue. A sip of water or a silent cough ("huh"—forceful burst of air with no voicing) are good alternatives.

- Frequent heartburn, a bitter taste in your mouth, or bad breath in the morning may be indicators of acid reflux, which may irritate your vocal folds and interfere with healthy singing. If you experience these symptoms, avoid eating late at night, go to bed with an empty stomach, eliminate spicy or high-acid foods, take a liquid antacid after meals and at bedtime, and elevate the head of your bed with blocks under the legs of the bed. If your symptoms persist, seek medical attention. You may need medication to reduce/ control the amount of stomach acid you produce.

- Sudden hoarseness can be an indicator of an acute vocal fold injury and should be taken very seriously. If you become hoarse suddenly, do not try to sing through it. Stop talking and singing. You need to be seen immediately by a laryngologist to be certain you are safe to continue singing/performing.

Emerich, K. & Sapir, S. 1999, November
Reprinted with permission.

**Voice Therapy—Plan of Treatment**

Patient:

Physician:

Diagnosis:            ICD-9:

Recommendation: _____ sessions of voice therapy

**Goals**

1. To improve phonation and reduce supraglottic adduction
2. To reduce laryngeal tension/hyperfunctional behaviors and improve overall vocal hygiene in order to reduce vocal pathology

**Objectives**

1. The patient will learn techniques to improve vocal hygiene and eliminate abusive vocal behaviors.
2. The patient will be provided with written information and neck/shoulder exercises to increase muscle awareness and relaxation of laryngeal and cervical tension.
3. The patient will learn diaphragmatic breathing techniques and methods of easy airflow release during speech.
4. The patient will engage in vocal exercises/practice to improve utilization of airflow.
5. The patient will improve self-monitoring of vocal quality, onset of phonation, pitch, volume, and laryngeal tension during conversational voice use.
6. The patient will engage in exercises to promote resonance and release of laryngeal tension.

**Progress**

Progress will be measured by acoustic and aerodynamic parameters within appropriate norms for age and sex. MPT and *s/z* ratio will be WNL. Reduction of laryngeal hyperfunction will be visually assessed (via videostroboscopic examination).

_____       _____

Speech-Language Pathologist                    Date

**Voice Therapy—Plan of Treatment**

Patient:

Physician:

Diagnosis: *s/p excision of vocal fold lesion*        ICD-9:

Recommendation: _____ sessions of voice therapy

## Goals

1. To improve phonation and restore vocal quality WFL (within functional limits)
2. To reduce laryngeal tension/hyperfunctional behaviors and improve overall vocal hygiene in order to inhibit recurrent vocal pathology

## Objectives

1. The patient will learn techniques to improve vocal hygiene and eliminate abusive vocal behaviors.
2. The patient will be provided with written information and neck/shoulder exercises to increase muscle awareness and relaxation of laryngeal and cervical tension.
3. The patient will learn diaphragmatic breathing techniques and methods of easy airflow release during speech.
4. The patient will engage in vocal exercises/practice to improve utilization of airflow.
5. The patient will improve self-monitoring of vocal quality, onset of phonation, pitch, volume, and laryngeal tension during conversational voice use.
6. The patient will engage in exercises to promote resonance and release of laryngeal tension.

## Progress

Progress will be measured by acoustic and aerodynamic parameters within appropriate norms for age and sex. MPT and *s/z* ratio will be WNL. Reduction of laryngeal hyperfunction and absence of recurrent pathology will be visually assessed (via videostroboscopic examination).

_____        _____
Speech-Language Pathologist                        Date

**Voice Therapy—Plan of Treatment**

Patient:

Physician:

Diagnosis:                    ICD-9:

Recommendations: _____ sessions of therapy

### Goals

1. To promote abduction of the true and/or false vocal folds
2. To promote relaxation of laryngeal structures for improved upper airway patency

### Objectives

1. The patient will learn techniques to promote diaphragmatic breath support.
2. The patient will learn techniques to improve utilization of airflow during breathing and speaking.
3. The patient will be provided with cervical exercises to improve muscle awareness and physical relaxation of cervical and laryngeal tension.
4. The patient will utilize breathing exercises and facilitative techniques to inhibit glottic/upper airway dysfunction.

### Progress

Progress will be measured by improvement in airflow and MPT measures and reduction of stridor (if present). Improved abduction and adduction during breathing and phonatory tasks will be assessed through laryngeal visualization.

_____                    _____

Speech-Language Pathologist                                    Date

**Voice Therapy—Plan of Treatment**

Patient:

Physician:

Diagnosis:                    ICD-9:

Recommendation: _____ sessions of voice therapy

### Goals
1. To improve overall laryngeal functioning for voice production, breathing, and/or swallowing.
2. To improve and maintain appropriate medial glottal closure upon phonation

### Objectives
1. The patient will learn techniques to improve vocal hygiene and maximize functioning without vocal hyperfunction/abuse.
2. The patient will engage in vocal exercises/practice to improve utilization of airflow during speech.
3. The patient will learn diaphragmatic breathing techniques and methods of easy airflow release.
4. The patient will engage in easy adduction exercises to improve medial glottal closure.
5. The patient will improve self-monitoring of vocal quality, onset of phonation, pitch, volume and laryngeal tension.
6. The patient will learn adaptive strategies utilizing head and neck positioning as needed to improve glottal closure.

### Progress
Progress will be measured by patient's ability to sustain phonation (MPT) and ability to achieve and maintain vocal parameters, including airflow measures that are WNL for patient's age and sex. Symptoms of dysphagia/aspiration (if present) will be reduced. Improvement of medial glottal closure will be assessed through visualization.

_____          _____
Speech-Language Pathologist                              Date

# 5 • HEAD AND NECK CANCER AND LARYNGECTOMY

*Head and neck cancer* is a term used to describe cancers of structures including the oral cavity, oropharynx, and larynx. This chapter provides basic medical, surgical, and therapeutic information to assist clinicians with assessment and rehabilitation of patients with various types of oral and laryngeal cancer. Continuing education and supervised clinical training is recommended.

## Your Role as Speech-Language Pathologist (SLP)

Your involvement in the evaluation and/or rehabilitation of patients with laryngeal cancers is a critical component of care. Your role focuses on speech, voice, and/or swallowing abilities that may have been surgically or functionally altered during the process of cancer treatment. Knowledge of medical treatment techniques and surgical procedures is essential to providing services to patients diagnosed with head and neck cancers.

Other members on the treatment team often include the following:

- otolaryngologist (ENT)
- medical oncologist
- radiation oncologist
- dentist/maxillofacial surgeon
- social worker

## Oral Cancer

Oral cancer may affect any part of the oral cavity, including the lips, tongue, gums (gingiva), cheeks (buccal mucosa), floor of the mouth, or palate (hard and soft). Changes in these structures or in their functions often result in speech and swallowing deficits. Since the voice remains intact in these patients, the following information serves as a brief outline of the facts about oral cancer, including diagnosis and treatment options.

### FACTS ABOUT ORAL CANCER

The most common form of oral cancer is squamous cell carcinoma (SCC).

#### Incidence

- 2-5% of all new cancers
- sixth most common malignancy in the world
- 30,000 new cases annually
- more common in men than women (2:1)
- typically appears between the ages of 50-70 years

The Source for Voice Disorders
Adolescent & Adult
Copyright © 2004 LinguiSystems, Inc.

## Risk factors

- cigarette, cigar, or pipe smoking
- smokeless tobacco ("snuff")
- alcohol abuse (considered a co-carcinogen along with smoking)
- poor oral hygiene

Recent advances in the diagnosis of oral cancer have identified the following as additional potential risk factors:

- previous malignancy
- vitamin/mineral deficiencies (riboflavin/iron)
- chemical/environmental exposure
- HIV, herpes, and immunodeficiency

## SYMPTOMS OF ORAL CANCER

- lump or thickening of oral tissue
- presence of a non-healing ulceration or lesion
- difficulty moving the tongue or jaw
- numbness of the tongue or other areas of the oral cavity
- swelling of oral structures
- loose teeth

## DIAGNOSIS OF ORAL CANCER

Early detection of oral cancer plays a critical role in curing the disease as well as preserving structures. The steps for oral examination should include the following:

- Remove any dentures or partial plates.
- Conduct a visual inspection of soft tissue. A whitish patch may represent leukoplakia and a reddish patch may represent erythroplakia.
- Palpate any visible lesions for changes in texture (firmness) and mobility (vs. fixed to surrounding tissues).
- Assess movement/identify restrictions in range of motion (ROM).
- Refer to ENT or dental professional for evaluation of lesions persisting longer than two weeks.

## TREATMENT OF ORAL CANCER

Oral cancers may be treated with surgery, radiation (XRT), or a combination of both. The surgical excision of structures most often involves a reconstruction of the oral cavity using skin grafts or muscular flaps to assist with both structure and function.

Chemotherapy has not been demonstrated to be effective alone; however, it may be used in conjunction with XRT (combination chemoradiation). This type of combination treatment has not demonstrated high success rates for cancers localized to the oral cavity (Suntharalingam et al. 2001), although it is used in higher stage, poor prognosis cancers. See pages 145-147 for side effects of radiation and chemotherapy treatment to the head/neck.

Cancer of the tongue (lingual carcinoma) often results in serious ramifications for speech and swallowing. Surgical excision (removal) of lingual carcinoma is called *partial* or *total glossectomy*.

Treatment after partial glossectomy may include the following:

- oral-motor exercises/range of movement (ROM)
- articulation (lingual productions most affected)
- improvement in palatal and pharyngeal compensation to reduce nasality resulting from altered oral space
- improvement in bolus manipulation for oral phase swallowing
- changes in position to improve swallowing
- changes in food texture/consistency for easier swallowing

Treatment after total glossectomy may involve the following:

- evaluation by a maxillofacial surgeon for prosthetic reconstruction
- swallowing evaluation to determine candidacy for return to oral feeding
  (*Note*:  Some patients may be unable to return to oral/PO feedings after total glossectomy.)
- Adaptive feeding utensils, changes in texture/consistency
- Slowed rate of speech with focus on labial productions

# Laryngeal Cancer

The following pages outline facts about laryngeal cancer, including diagnosis and treatment information.

## FACTS ABOUT LARYNGEAL CANCER

### Incidence

- 10,000 new cases per year
- greater than 90% are squamous cell carcinomas (SCC)
- typically occurs between the ages of 50-70 years
- more common in men than women (4:1)

### Risk factors

- smoking
- alcohol consumption
- environmental (e.g., chemical or toxin exposure)
- family history

There is a synergistic effect of the above risk factors—a combination of these risk factors poses a greater risk than each factor individually.

Laryngeal cancers are divided into the following categories:

- supraglottic
- glottic
- subglottic

The following pages will provide descriptions and symptoms of tumors within the supraglottic, glottic, and subglottic regions and the tumor or *T* classification of each. This information will help you understand the structures involved with a particular tumor.

## SUPRAGLOTTIC CANCER

Supraglottic cancer may involve any of the following structures:

- epiglottis
- false vocal folds (FVFs)
- ventricles
- aryepiglottic folds
- arytenoids

Symptoms associated with supraglottic cancer may include the sensation of a lump in the throat, pain referred to the ear, and dysphagia or odynophagia (pain upon swallowing), which may result in weight loss.

### Tumor Staging

| | |
|---|---|
| T1 | tumor limited to one site of the supraglottis with normal vocal fold (VF) mobility |
| T2 | tumor invades more than one site of the supraglottis or glottis with normal VF mobility |
| T3 | tumor limited to the larynx with VF fixation and/or invasion of the postcricoid area, medial wall of the pyriform sinuses, or pre-epiglottic space |
| T4 | tumor invasion through the thyroid cartilage, and/or extends to the other tissues beyond the larynx (e.g., oropharynx, soft tissue of the neck) |

## GLOTTIC CANCER

Glottic cancer involves the true vocal folds/glottis.

Symptoms of glottic cancer include hoarseness, airway obstruction/stridor, and coughing/throat-clearing.

### Tumor Staging

| | |
|---|---|
| T1 | tumor limited to the VFs (may invade the anterior or posterior commissure) with normal VF mobility |
| T1a | tumor limited to one VF |
| T1b | tumor involves both VFs |
| T2 | tumor extends to supra and/or subglottis with impaired VF mobility |

T3    tumor limited to VFs with fixation

T4    tumor invasion through the thyroid cartilage and/or extension to tissues beyond the larynx (e.g., oropharynx, soft tissue of the neck)

## SUBGLOTTIC CANCER

Subglottic cancer may involve the cricoid cartilage and upper airway.

Patients are often asymptomatic until later stages. This is dangerous because there are no early warning signs. When symptoms do occur, they most often include hoarseness and airway obstruction.

## Tumor Staging

T1    tumor limited to the subglottis

T2    tumor extends to the VFs

T3    tumor confined to the larynx with VF fixation

T4    tumor invades the cricoid and/or thyroid and invades other tissues beyond the larynx (e.g., oropharynx, soft tissue of the neck)

## OVERALL TUMOR STAGING FOR LARYNGEAL CANCER

Cancer is "staged" in order to define the extent and severity of the tumor. The TNM system (tumor, nodes, metastasis) is used to report the stage of the cancer. The *T* identifies the site and size of the tumor with T4 representing a large tumor involving the entire structure. *N* classification indicates the size of metastatic lymph nodes within the neck (N0–N3). *N0* indicates the absence of positive nodes and *N3* represents severe lymph node involvement. *M* classification indicates the presence of distant metastasis (M0–M3). *M0* indicates the absence of metastasis from the primary site of the larynx and *M3* indicates significant involvement of a distant site (e.g., lungs, brain).

The TNM classification provides an overall "stage" of the disease to assist in the physician's/surgeon's choice of treatment and determines the prognosis for cure. (See treatment section, page 145.)

*Note*: Pre-cancerous lesions are referred to as *carcinoma in situ*.

| Stage | TNM classification |
|-------|--------------------|
| I | T1, N0, M0 |
| II | T2, N0, M0 |
| III | T3, N0, MO<br>T1-T3, N1, M0 |
| IV | T4, N0-N1, M0<br>T1-T4, N2-N3, M0<br>T1-T4, N0-N3, M1 |

## DIAGNOSIS

A diagnosis of laryngeal cancer is made by a physician after a thorough history of the problem, head and neck examination, visual inspection of the larynx, and further medical work-up that may include the following procedures:

- CT scan/MRI
- chest X-ray
- complete blood count (CBC)
- biopsy of lesion via direct laryngoscopy (performed by ENT)

Early detection of laryngeal cancer results in possible treatment without surgery (i.e., radiation), thereby preserving structure and maintaining the patient's ability to phonate and swallow.

## TREATMENT

Treatment for laryngeal cancer may be medical and/or surgical and may include radiation therapy (XRT), chemotherapy (in combination with radiation therapy), and/or surgical excision to remove the lesion/site and neck dissection if positive nodes are identified (see Radical Neck Dissection, page 149).

The following are terms often used to describe the type of medical/surgical treatment:

**Organ preservation:** the ability to treat cancer with radiation alone or in combination with chemotherapy, eliminating the need for surgical excision and thereby preserving laryngeal structures

**Surgical salvage:** surgical excision of involved structures when radiation and/or chemoradiation fails to eliminate the tumor

**Surgical conservation:** surgical removal of the cancer while preserving uninvolved structures

As mentioned above, the type of treatment chosen is often based on the stage of the cancer. Therefore, the cure rate associated with medical/surgical intervention is influenced by factors such as the location and size of the tumor, infiltration to other structures, the presence of cancerous lymph nodes, and metastasis (spread to distant sites).

## Radiation Therapy

The following section is designed to provide information about treatment of head and neck cancer with radiation (XRT). Knowledge of the potential side effects from radiation treatment to the head and neck will help you make appropriate therapeutic recommendations and counseling for patients undergoing XRT.

## Side Effects of Radiation Treatment to the Head and Neck

Side effects may include the following:

- skin rash ("radiation burn")
- sore throat
- hoarseness
- possible breathing difficulty
- dysphagia/odynophagia
- fatigue
- mucositis/mouth sores
- trismus (spasm of muscles used in mastication)

With radiation treatment, the tissue of the neck may also become tender, swollen, hardened (fibrosis), and may potentially break down (necrosis/radionecrosis). Bone loss may also occur (osteoradionecrosis).

Radiation to lymph nodes located near salivary glands results in permanent "dry mouth" (xerostomia) from the reduction of saliva. In turn, less saliva and potential bone loss often result in permanent tooth decay, so many patients undergo removal of some or all of their teeth prior to radiation treatment. Patients who do not undergo dental extractions should be encouraged to receive dental care and fluoride treatments throughout the course of radiation.

The following are symptoms that patients may experience while undergoing radiation treatment. The recommendations have been adapted from the American Cancer Society's *CancerCare* Series on Nutrition, Symptoms, and Solutions.

## Dry Mouth/Dehydration

This condition is evidenced by cotton mouth, dry oral mucosa and lips, weakness, dizziness, and reduced urination.

*Recommendations*
- Increase fluids (if patient is cleared for liquids by mouth).
- Provide ice chips (if patient is cleared for liquids by mouth).
- Encourage sugar-free hard candy.
- Use petroleum-based jelly on lips.
- Use a humidifier.
- Try a saliva substitute or artificial saliva.

## Mouth Sores

Mouth sores are evidenced by mouth tenderness, sores or lesions in the mouth, bleeding from oral mucosa, and cracked or bleeding lips.

*Recommendations*
- Use petroleum-based jelly on lips.
- Avoid mouthwash containing alcohol.
- Rinse mouth (may use combination of salt and water or baking soda and water).
- Avoid toothpicks, toothbrushes, and dental floss if they cause discomfort (use cotton or sponge swabs to clean mouth/teeth).
- Eat soft foods.
- Avoid citrus and spicy foods.

## Changes in Smell and Taste, Appetite Change, and Weight Loss

These changes are evidenced by decreased appetite, upset stomach from food odors, food tasting different, weight loss, and feeling full fast (i.e., inability to eat normal portions).

*Recommendations*
- Eat 3-4 hours ahead of treatments.
- Eat light meals more frequently and/or snack throughout the day.
- Eat $\frac{1}{3}$ of your calories in the morning (breakfast) because appetite deteriorates during the day.
- Include high protein/high calorie foods in your diet (e.g., whole milk, cheese, peanut butter).
- Avoid cooking foods with strong odors and/or eat cold foods.
- Keep mouth fresh and clean by frequent rinsing.

## Vocal Effects of Radiation Therapy

Radiation effects to the larynx include edema/swelling of laryngeal structures, dryness of the vocal fold mucosa, and stiffness of the vocal fold mucosal covering. As a result, patients with laryngeal cancer treated with radiation therapy often experience changes in vocal quality during and after radiation. The vocal changes may include hoarseness, reduction of pitch, and strained vocalization.

In cases of significant laryngeal edema, patients may exhibit stridor that should be closely monitored to ensure an open airway. In some cases, patients will require a tracheostomy.

Due to the inflammation of the larynx and vocal folds during the course of radiation therapy, vocal rest and increased hydration should be encouraged. Patients should not engage in strenuous vocal use or demanding vocal exercise. Instead, encourage relaxed vocalization practice to maintain vocal flexibility during this time.

Recommendations may include the following exercises:
- humming—easy relaxed humming to elicit vocal fold vibration
- pitch scales/glides—Have the patient hum or produce low-pitched and high-pitched vowel sounds; use pitch scales from lower to higher pitches.
- vocal function exercises (page 91)

## Chemotherapy

If the patient is also receiving chemotherapy, the side effects noted for radiation therapy may be more severe, including:

- skin rash ("radiation burn")
- sore throat
- hoarseness
- possible breathing difficulty
- dysphagia/odynophagia
- fatigue

In addition, chemotherapy may also cause nausea, vomiting, diarrhea, and constipation. Recommendations may include smaller, low-fat meals; reduction of dairy products; and refraining from eating one or two hours prior to XRT or chemotherapy.

## Surgical Management of Laryngeal Cancers

The following sections review surgical procedures most often associated with the treatment of laryngeal cancer. These procedures may vary slightly, depending upon the invasion of the cancer to surrounding structures. With the development of new laser surgical techniques and robot assisted surgeries, there has been reported improvement in overall patient outcomes, including avoidance of tracheostomy; less recovery time; and better preservation of speech, voice, and swallow function.

An operative report is useful to provide information regarding the extent of structures excised as well as any reconstructive procedures performed. Each procedure is defined in terms of structural excision and follow-up rehabilitation needed by the SLP.

## Total Laryngectomy

In a total laryngectomy, the entire larynx, including the hyoid bone, is removed. The trachea is directed forward and sutured to the skin to create a stoma. The pharynx and esophagus remain intact for swallowing.

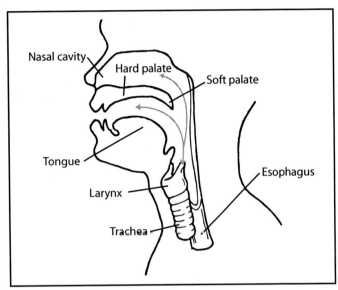

Figure 26.  Before laryngectomy

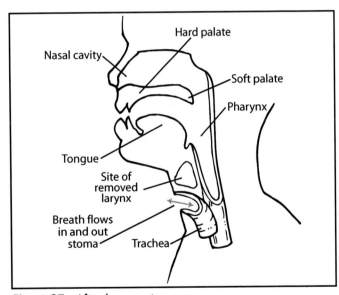

Figure 27.  After laryngectomy

Additional surgical procedures may be needed if evidence is found of the cancer invading surrounding structures. These include the following:

- pharyngo-laryngectomy
- esophageal resection
- composite resection
- radical neck dissection

Cancer extending to the pharynx or esophagus may require a *pharyngo-laryngectomy* and/or *esophageal resection*. In these procedures, portions of the pharynx and/or esophagus are removed in addition to a total laryngectomy. Reconstruction may involve a gastric pull-up (esophagus is pulled superiorly) or a jejunal interposition (a section of the small intestine called the *jejunum* is used to reconstruct the pharyngo-esophageal segment), or muscular flap reconstruction (e.g., pectoralis muscle).

These procedures may reduce the functional ability to use esophageal or tracheo-esophageal speech, creating a "tight" and/or "wet" vocal quality. These patients may experience swallowing difficulties and need to remain on soft or pureed foods or require frequent alternation of liquids to assist in bolus transport.

In a *composite resection* (also called a commando), several structures of the head and neck may be removed in addition to the larynx secondary to spread or metastasis. These may include the palate, base of the tongue, floor of the mouth, and mandible.

In a *radical neck dissection* (RND) the lymphatic system on one or both sides of the neck may be removed to eliminate evidence of cancer spread to the lymph nodes. Metastasis to the lymph nodes increases with the size of the tumor.

---

*Important Facts for Clinicians*

Clinicians working with the rehabilitation of laryngectomy patients should keep in mind the following anatomical and functional changes:

- loss of voice (need to develop an alternate means of communication)
- airway is separated from the nose and mouth (can no longer breathe through nose/mouth)
- stoma should remain widely patent (open) but should be protected from environmental elements
- swallowing should remain intact (aspiration is only a concern in the presence of a fistula [hole] between the trachea and esophagus)

---

# Laryngectomy Facts for the Patient

This information sheet can be used for pre/post-operative counseling to provide patients and caregivers with the basic facts about the changes associated with a laryngectomy.

*Stoma* = opening in your neck through which you breathe

1. Since you no longer breathe through your nose or mouth, your senses of smell and taste are diminished or absent.

2. You will be unable to blow your nose or sneeze.

3. Use humidification to reduce dryness.

4. When coughing, you should cover your stoma (not your mouth) as this is now the opening through which you will expel air, foreign material, or phlegm/mucous.

5. You will be unable to hold your breath or "bear down," making it difficult to lift heavy objects.

## Protection of your stoma

1. You will need to protect your stoma from foreign material. Use stoma shields and covers made of breathable material.

2. Protect your stoma from water entering into your lungs.
   Use a shower guard or shower protector.
   Do not go swimming or engage in water sports.

## Important Notes

Wear a MedicAlert bracelet and use an ID card in your wallet and/or sticker in your car to let others know that you are a "neck breather." These items are available through the American Cancer Society.

***CPR rescue breathing must be performed via your stoma to direct air into your lungs.

## Partial Laryngectomy

The following surgical procedures involve organ conservation as they maintain the integrity of uninvolved laryngeal structures to allow for rehabilitation of phonation and swallowing. These procedures *do not* involve the creation of a stoma:

- vertical hemilaryngectomy
- supraglottic laryngectomy
- supracricoid partial laryngectomy

### Vertical Hemilaryngectomy

The larynx is surgically divided at or near midline (vertically) to remove the tumor. Structures removed on the involved side include the thyroid lamina, arytenoid, true vocal fold, and often the false vocal fold. Surgical reconstruction often includes the creation of a neoglottis (newly created "glottis" or vibratory segment) using pharyngeal or muscular flaps.

After this surgery, the patient phonates by adducting the one functioning vocal fold and arytenoid to contact the newly created contralateral wall. Therapy may include the use of head rotation to the resected (removed) side to improve closure for vibratory phonation and for swallowing. Therapy tasks may also include the use of forced or "pushed" phonation. See adduction exercises (pages 101-102).

### Supraglottic Laryngectomy

Structures above the glottis are removed (horizontal excision), including the ventricular folds, aryepiglottic folds, epiglottis, hyoid, and/or the superior portions of the thyroid cartilage.

Vocal quality remains intact in these patients. The focus of therapeutic rehabilitation is swallowing and the use of supraglottic swallowing techniques to prevent aspiration. (See Logemann 1998.)

### Supracricoid Partial Laryngectomy (SCPL)

The following acronyms are commonly used to distinguish the extent of structural excision and reconstruction used during the surgical procedure.

- SCPL-CHEP: supracricoid partial laryngectomy-cricohyoidoepiglottopexy
- SCPL-CHP: supracricoid partial laryngectomy-cricohyoidopexy

These procedures involve surgical excision (horizontal) for removal of structures above the cricoid cartilage, including the true vocal folds and sometimes the entire epiglottis (CHP). The procedure *must* preserve the cricoid, hyoid, and at least one arytenoid. The remaining arytenoid is surgically pulled anteriorly and laterally to assist in achieving closure for voice and swallowing.

The patient will need to undergo rehabilitation of both speech and swallowing by learning forceful adduction techniques of the remaining arytenoid(s) (e.g., pulling, pages 101-102) to produce supraglottic voicing and use of effortful/pushed phonation.  You can address swallowing by using supraglottic swallow techniques.  (See Logemann 1998.)

# Evaluation and Counseling

A large part of your pre-operative and post-operative evaluation involves counseling and provision of information to the patient and caregivers.  This counseling is to provide support needed to deal with the physical changes, as well as encouragement for developing effective alaryngeal communication.

## PRE-OPERATIVE EVALUATION AND COUNSELING

The following is a general outline to help you obtain information that will assist in post-operative treatment for return to functional communication.

### Evaluation

**Assess patient's communication needs.**
- Living situation—What is the patient's need for communication within his home environment?
- Occupation—What is the patient's need for communication within his work environment?  Does the patient intend to return to work?
- Social requirements—What are other social communication needs (e.g., worship, travel)?
- Hobbies—Does the patient have a hobby that requires use of his voice?

**Screen/evaluate baseline communication skills in the following areas:**
- Cognitive status—ability to understand and participate in rehabilitation process
- Articulation—intelligibility
- Language—receptive and expressive language skills
- Voice—volume and respiratory parameters
- Rate—rate of speech
- Fluency—presence of/severity of dysfluency
- Reading/writing skills—Are they functional for communication?
- Hearing—presence of a hearing loss

**Obtain the following information from the referring physician:**
- What type of surgical excision is to be performed?
- Has the patient had radiation?  Will the patient be undergoing radiation post-operatively?

### Counseling

A pre-operative counseling session should incorporate the following information:
- First review what the patient has already been told by his physician.
- Find out what treatments the patient has already undergone.
- Address any misunderstandings or concerns.
- Provide new information (written when possible).
- Discuss post-operative course of treatment and what to expect.

Keep in mind the *amount* of information you provide the patient/family/caregiver. They may or may not be able to comprehend too much or too detailed information at this time. Make clinical judgments about information to present based on the questions they ask.

The type of information and the way it is presented to the patient varies from physician to physician. Be aware of the clinical practice patterns of referring physicians and tailor the information you present to how that physician prefers to proceed with medical and surgical treatment. A consistency in presentation and positive attitude regarding outcomes will reinforce the patient's confidence in his surgeon/doctor.

## POST-OPERATIVE EVALUATION AND COUNSELING

Provide the patient with a means to communicate in the immediate post-operative period when voicing will not be possible (e.g., written, communication board). The pre-operative assessment regarding communication needs and baseline speech, language, and cognitive status will help you choose an optimal post-operative communication mode.

Post-operative counseling may address the following emotional issues, both with the patient and family/support system. A social worker plays a critical role in this period of rehabilitation.

- fear of cancer survival and the identification of oneself as a "cancer survivor"
- dealing with physical changes in appearance/self image
- accepting the loss of voice
- social implications/dealing with the reactions of others
- economic concerns related to medical bills, equipment, and supplies

Support groups and programs offer a variety of organized programs for patients and families and should be encouraged in the post-operative period. (See Resources: Organizations and Support Groups, page 169.)

Make sure the patient and his family has contact information for you or for the clinician who will follow him after surgery, as well as for the social worker assigned to the patient's case.

Provide the patient with written information and resources to obtain medical supplies such as stoma covers, shower guards, and electrolarynx or tracheo-esophageal puncture (TEP) supplies. (See Resources, page 168.)

# Rehabilitation

As discussed in Chapter 1, there are three components to voice production:

Respiration = power source (air)
Phonation = sound generator (vocal folds)
Resonance = resonator/filter (head/neck)

Even with an altered anatomical structure, there are several ways for a person with a laryngectomy to

The Source for Voice Disorders
Adolescent & Adult
Copyright © 2004 LinguiSystems, Inc.

produce voicing. The following is a brief overview of the speaking options and corresponding therapy tasks that are available to laryngectomized patients.

These methods include:
- esophageal speech
- use of an electrolarynx
- tracheo-esophageal speech

## ESOPHAGEAL SPEECH

One of the oldest and non-invasive ways of achieving post-laryngectomy voicing is esophageal speech. This voicing technique is accomplished by injecting air into the esophagus and releasing it, thereby vibrating the pharyngeal-esophageal segment in order to promote generation of sound. (See Figure 28.)

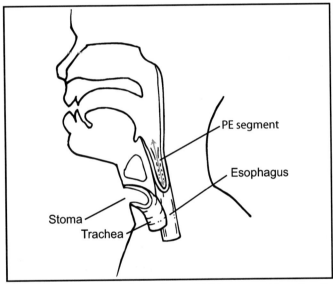

Figure 28. Pharyngeal-esophageal (PE) segment for vibration

There are various ways to inject air into the esophagus. This type of training is provided in speech therapy. Some examples are the injection method, the swallow method, and the inhalation method.

**injection method**: Air is injected into the upper esophagus through the use of intraoral pressure that is built up and then directed backward with the tongue.

**swallow method**: Air is swallowed into the esophagus and then immediately released back into the mouth.

**inhalation method**: The mouth is opened and the pharynx relaxed as air is inhaled into the upper esophagus.

The patient's ability to become proficient in these methods can impact the naturalness of phrasing and fluency of running speech. Clinician instruction is also necessary to practice the timing/phrasing for airflow release and the articulatory shaping of sounds. Recommendations for therapy are listed on the next page.

## Treatment Tasks

- find the optimal method for air injection into the esophagus for each individual patient (page 155)
- practice multisyllabic words (page 161)
- social phrases (page 160) to practice intelligibility for frequently used conversational phrases
- conversational speech practice

### USE OF AN ELECTROLARYNX

An electrolarynx acts as a sound generator by providing vibration to the oropharyngeal cavity. To do so, the patient uses an adapter placed in the mouth (intraoral) or places the electrolarynx on soft tissue, most commonly on the neck. In some instances, intraoral adapters may be preferred immediately after surgery because of the tenderness of neck tissue and surgical staples/stitches. Once the vibration is transmitted into the pharyngeal or oral cavity, the patient shapes it into speech by using the articulators (lips, teeth, tongue). Most electrolarynx devices are battery operated and the specific features vary according to each individual brand/model. (See Resources, page 167, for suppliers and distributors.)

The following guidelines are important when instructing a patient on electrolarynx use:

- Use the non-dominant hand to allow for multitasking when speaking.
- When an intraoral adapter is used, place the adapter in the farthest position in the corner of the mouth in order to minimize interference with the articulators during continuous speech production.
- For neck placement, place the electrolarynx on the "soft" tissue of the neck in order to optimize vibratory conduction. Use buccal placement (against the cheek) if severe fibrosis of the neck inhibits vibration.
- Only deliver vibration when articulating a word/phrase. Let go of the button between words/phrases.
- Over-articulate or use exaggerated tongue and lip movements for better understanding.

## Treatment Tasks

- placement of the electrolarynx (e.g., intraoral, soft tissue) as noted above
- maintenance and troubleshooting of the device itself
- adjustment of pitch/volume controls
- delivery/timing of vibration with verbalizations
- practice multisyllabic words (page 161)
- social phrases (page 160) to practice intelligibility for frequently used conversational phrases
- conversational speech practice

### TRACHEOESOPHAGEAL SPEECH

Tracheoesophageal speech is quickly becoming the method of choice for many laryngectomees. The vocal quality produced is similar to that of traditional esophageal speech; however, the method for air injection makes it unique. Tracheoesophageal speech restores use of the lungs as the driving power for voice production.

156

Tracheoesophageal speech requires a surgical procedure. The otolaryngologist (ENT) creates a puncture through the posterior wall of the trachea into the esophagus, restoring communication between the airway and the pharynx/oral cavities. (See Figure 29.) This puncture is called a *tracheo-esophageal fistula* or *tracheo-esophageal puncture* (TEP). The puncture may be made at the time of the laryngectomy surgery (primary placement) or during a subsequent surgery at any time following a total laryngectomy (secondary placement).

In cases of secondary TEP placement, the SLP may be asked to perform an insufflation test, which is a procedure involving the placement of a catheter through the patient's nose (transnasal) with a housing attached to the peri-stomal area (around the perimeter of the stoma). This allows for delivery of air injection from the patient's airway (stoma) through the catheter to the PE segment to assess vibration and ability to produce esophageal voice. A positive insufflation test produces voice and reveals the patient is a good candidate for placement of a TEP.

Following the surgical procedure, a one-way prosthetic valve is placed to keep the fistula open and to direct air into the esophagus. Use of a one-way valve prevents aspiration of liquids/food into back into the trachea. Upon occlusion of the stoma (Figure 30), air is directed into the esophagus to vibrate the pharyngo-esophageal segment for voicing.

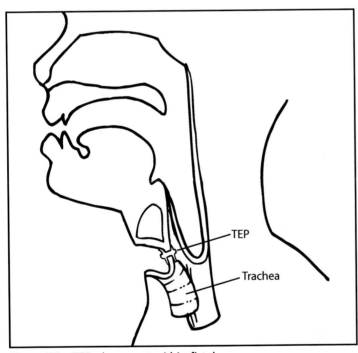

Figure 29. TEP placement within fistula

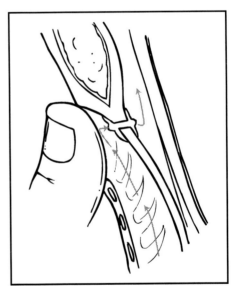

Figure 30. Occlusion of stoma

In most instances, SLPs are responsible for:

- insufflation test (if secondary puncture)
- sizing the puncture tract
- choosing the correct length/diameter of prosthesis
- fitting, placement, and changing of prosthesis
- patient education regarding maintenance of prosthesis

*Special Note*:  In order to provide safe and adequate care for TEP patients, it is necessary to obtain "hands-on" training with proper supervision prior to attempting to fit, place, or change a TE prosthesis. Intervention with this patient population should only be performed in a medical setting that has the necessary tools and equipment to adequately complete TEP sizing and placement.

Placement of a valve is not permanent.  Changing of the prosthesis is required by either the SLP or, in some cases, the patient and/or caregivers trained in the procedure.  Indications for prosthesis change include the following:

- leaking of liquids through or around the valve
- loss of voicing ability
- pistoning (anterior/posterior movement) of the valve within the puncture tract, if the valve is too long

The average life of a prosthesis varies from three to six months, depending on the type of valve and care of the valve.  Premature failure of the valve can occur due to candida (yeast) growth on the prosthesis or formation of granulation tissue surrounding the puncture.  (See page 162 for troubleshooting guidelines.)

## Treatment Tasks

- instruction regarding prosthesis care and cleaning of the valve
- emergency procedures in case the valve becomes dislodged
- provision of ordering information for additional tracheostoma accessories (Resources, page 168)
- stomal occlusion—use of finger occlusion or other "hands-free" options (see below)
- breathing and stomal occlusion practice to coordinate exhalation and phonation
- multisyllable words (page 160)
- contrastive drills emphasizing use of varying volumes—practice "soft" (less push of airflow) vs. "loud" (increased airflow) phonation

In addition to the above treatment tasks, a number of devices can be provided and demonstrated to patients using TEP speech.  These devices include a hands-free device or tracheostoma valve, which allows the patient to speak without manual occlusion of the stoma.  These also can be used with housing devices to assist in humidification of the stoma.  These devices may be obtained through distributors listed in Resources, page 168.

# Pros and Cons of Speech Options

| | Esophageal Speech | Use of Electrolarynx | Tracheoesophageal Speech |
|---|---|---|---|
| **Pros** | hands-free system (doesn't require stomal occlusion)<br><br>no costly speech devices<br><br>no maintenance<br><br>relatively natural speech quality<br><br>always available and ready for use | can be used immediately following surgery for communication<br><br>easy to learn<br><br>good "back-up" communication system (even if patient has a TEP)<br><br>non-invasive | relatively natural voice quality<br><br>always accessible<br><br>hands-free accessories available (Manual stoma occlusion is not the only option.) |
| **Cons** | requires a time commitment for therapy<br><br>difficult to learn<br><br>difficult to find a qualified clinician for instruction<br><br>reduced fluency of speech | poor quality/unnatural—may not be considered socially acceptable<br><br>restricts mobility (occupies the use of a hand for placement/use)<br><br>expensive<br><br>equipment maintenance, battery replacement, and repair if needed | requires surgical creation of puncture<br><br>expensive supplies<br><br>risk of aspiration of the prosthesis<br><br>requires maintenance and changing of the valve<br><br>occasional leaking of liquids/aspiration<br><br>increased risk of granulation tissue |

Hello.

Good-bye.

Good luck.

Go home.

Please.

Thank you.

Hurry up.

See you soon.

Come back later.

Happy Birthday.

Welcome home.

How are you?

Where are you going?

What time is it?

Leave me alone.

Who is it?

What is your name?

I need help.

I need an appointment.

Wash the dishes.

I need a drink.

Pay the bills.

Call the doctor.

Pass the salt.

I am cold.

I am fine.

I do not know.

I feel sick.

The Source for Voice Disorders
Adolescent & Adult
Copyright © 2004 LinguiSystems, Inc.

| | |
|---|---|
| university | rehabilitation |
| refrigerator | professional |
| immediately | electrician |
| photography | hippopotamus |
| kindergarten | terrifying |
| cafeteria | politically |
| impossibility | ballerina |
| dictionary | humidity |
| Yugoslavia | adolescent |
| motorcycle | misunderstanding |
| encyclopedia | reliability |
| pediatrician | sophistication |
| medication | identification |
| difficulty | transportation |

# Troubleshooting Chart for Tracheoesophageal Puncture and Prosthesis Problems

| Problem | Causes | Solutions |
|---|---|---|
| Leakage *through* prosthesis | 1. Duckbill tip contact against posterior esophageal wall<br>2. Valve deterioration<br>3. Candida deposits on/in valve mechanism | 1. Replace with low pressure type prosthesis.<br>2. Replace prosthesis.<br>3. Regular prosthesis disinfection in hydrogen peroxide |
| Leakage *around* prosthesis | 1. Prosthesis is too long, resulting in piston movement/tract dilation.<br>2. Insufficient tracheoesophageal party wall thickness<br>3. Irradiated tissue | 1. Resize to a shorter prosthesis.<br>2. Reconstruct tracheoesophageal party wall with muscle flap.<br>3. Flap reconstruction |
| Microstoma | 1. Stenosis | 1. a) Silicone tracheostoma vent<br>b) Surgical revision of tracheostoma (enlargement) |
| Macrostoma | 1. Natural trachea size/tracheomalacia | 1. Surgical revision of tracheostoma (reduction) |
| Granulation tissue formation | 1. Irritation/inflammation/tissue thickness (circumferential "donut") associated with presence of foreign body | 1. a) Surgical removal of tissue (circumferential "donut")<br>b) Increase frequency of prosthesis removal and disinfection. |
| *Immediate* post-fitting aphonia/dysphonia | 1. Prosthesis valved tip is stuck secondary to increased saliva viscosity.<br>2. Forceful stoma occlusion<br>3. Pharyngeal constrictor spasm | 1. Remove prosthesis and inspect valve. Lubricate valve mechanism with vegetable oil (cooking oil).<br>2. Light finger contact<br>3. a) Assess voicing without prosthesis.*<br>b) Transtracheal insufflation via 18FR catheter<br>c) Insufflation under fluoroscopy*<br>d) Pharyngeal plexus nerve block* |
| *Delayed* post-fitting aphonia/dysphonia | 1. Failure to fully insert prosthesis<br>2. Puncture tract closure secondary to inadequate prosthesis length<br>3. Prosthesis valved tip is stuck. | 1. Dilate and re-insert prosthesis.<br>2. Dilate and re-insert longer prosthesis.<br>3. Remove prosthesis and inspect valve. Lubricate valve with vegetable oil. |
| Insufficient tracheostoma valve tape seal duration | 1. Excessive system back pressure<br><br>2. Failure to cleanse skin prior to valve placement<br>3. Failure to allow adhesive to dry<br>4. Careless application/use | 1. a) Assess intertracheal pressure during connected speech with pressure meter.<br>b) Alter prosthesis type/diameter.<br>c) Reduce speech loudness.<br>2. a) Clean skin with alcohol.<br>b) Cleanse adhesive solvent from skin surface with alcohol.<br>3. Wait 3-4 minutes before applying tape housing to adhesive coated skin.<br>4. a) Reinstruct in method of application.<br>b) Remove valve prior to coughing. |

Reprinted from Blom, E., Hamaker, R., & Freeman, S. (1994). Postlaryngectomy voice restoration. In Frank E. Lucente, M.D. (Ed.), *Highlights of the Instructional Courses*, 7, 9, with permission from Elsevier

\* Pharyngeal constrictor myotomy if fluent voicing can't be achieved

# GLOSSARY

| | |
|---|---|
| **abduction** | open; away from midline |
| **acoustic analysis** | properties of a sound wave analyzed instrumentally |
| **adduction** | closed; toward midline |
| **amplitude/intensity** | perceptual correlate is volume or loudness; also called *energy*; measured by the amplitude or magnitude of the sound wave generated in decibels (dB) |
| **amplitude** | the extent of horizontal excursion of the vocal folds during movement |
| **anterior** | from the front |
| **autologous fat** | fat taken from one spot on a person's body to be used elsewhere in the body |
| **aphonia** | absence of voice; no vibratory voicing |
| **aphonic breaks** | a break or interruption in the vibration/phonation |
| **breathy** | audible escape of air; a weak vocal tone; glottal insufficiency |
| **clavicular breathing** | use of upper chest and shoulder muscles with excessive movement during inspiration |
| **contralateral** | on the opposite side of the body |
| **Cushing's syndrome** | syndrome caused by excessive production of the adrenal or pituitary gland, resulting in obesity and muscular weakness |
| **diaphragmatic breathing** | use of the diaphragm to produce an outward movement of the abdomen in inhalation; optimal breathing pattern for speech/singing |
| **diplophonia** | the presence of two tones or pitches heard simultaneously during phonation |
| **dyskinesia** | impaired control of voluntary movement |
| **dysphonia** | an abnormal vocal quality |
| **EGG** | produces a visual representation (waveform) of the ratio of open phase to closed phase during the glottic cycle and is used as a technique to assess vocal fold contact |
| **expiratory reserve volume (ERV)** | the maximum volume that can be expired beyond spontaneous or tidal expiration (1500-2000cc) |
| **focal** | concentrated within a small area |
| **frequency** | perceptual correlate is pitch; measured in cycles per second (Hertz/Hz) |

| | |
|---|---|
| **fundamental frequency** | the lowest frequency of first harmonic of the voice correlating to a physical measure of vocal fold vibration |
| **glottal attack** | hyperadduction of the vocal folds at the onset of phonation |
| **glottal fry** | pulse register; use of the lowest register during phonation; increased closed phase of the vibratory cycle |
| **glottic closure** | the degree that the vocal folds approximate during the closed phase of vibration |
| **glottis** | the space between the vocal folds |
| **harmonics** | multiples of the fundamental frequency |
| **harsh** | irregular vocal fold vibrations; a "raspy" or unmusical tone; a combination of hoarse and breathy |
| **Hashimoto's** | chronic inflammation of the thyroid characterized by goiter or thyroid fibrosis |
| **hoarseness** | excessive "noise" in the signal; an unpleasant, rough vocal quality |
| **hyperfunction** | increased supraglottic tension or the presence of false fold adduction |
| **hyperfunctional** | excessive muscular effort; over exertion |
| **hypofunctional** | reduced function; low muscular effort |
| **hyperkinesia** | increase in movement resulting in spasticity or tremor |
| **hypokinesia** | reduction of movement resulting in rigidity |
| **hypernasality** | excessive nasality; increased sound diverted into the nasal airway |
| **hyponasality** | insufficient nasality; denasal; reduction in nasal resonance |
| **inferior** | from below |
| **inspiratory reserve volume (IRV)** | the volume of air that can be inspired after normal tidal inspiration (1500-2500cc) |
| **ipsalateral** | on the same side of the body |
| **jitter** | a short-term cycle-to-cycle variation in fundamental frequency detected during a sustained vowel; a measure of instability from cycle to cycle in the vibratory characteristics of the vocal folds |
| **laterally** | away from midline |

The Source for Voice Disorders
Adolescent & Adult
Copyright © 2004 LinguiSystems, Inc.

| | |
|---|---|
| **lupus** | any of several inflammatory diseases characterized by skin lesions |
| **medialization thyroplasty** | a surgical procedure used to medialize the vocal folds |
| **medially** | toward midline |
| **metastasis** | the transfer of disease to another part of the body |
| **MPT** | an estimated measure of airflow during voicing |
| **mucosal wave** | the mucosa traveling over the body from the medial edge to half the width of the true vocal fold |
| **noise** | aperiodic or random distribution of acoustical energy |
| **paramedian** | slightly lateral of midline; slightly abducted position |
| **partial glossectomy** | surgical resection of a portion of the tongue |
| **pemphagoid** | a disease resulting in inflammation/eruptions of skin and mucous membranes |
| **perichondrium** | a fibrous connective tissue membrane of cartilage |
| **periodicity** | the regularity of successive cycles of vibration |
| **perturbation** | a disturbance in the regularity of the waveform that correlates to perceived roughness or harshness |
| **pharyngeal constrictor myotomy** | surgical incision to divide or release muscular fibers of the pharyngeal complex |
| **pitch breaks** | an interruption in the frequency of vibration (a voice can break up or down in pitch); a shift in vocal register during singing |
| **polycondritis** | a degenerative disease characterized by recurrent inflammation of the cartilage in the body |
| **posterior** | from the back |
| **presbylarynx** | physiological changes to the vocal fold(s), resulting in atrophy/bowing of the muscle |
| **proximal** | toward the center of the body |
| **resection** | the surgical removal of a structure |
| **residual volume (RV)** | the volume of gas/air remaining in the lungs after maximum expiration; the residual lung volume that cannot be expelled (1000-1500cc) |

| | |
|---|---|
| *s/z* ratio | a comparative measure of a voiceless/voiced cognate pair |
| shimmer | a short-term cycle-to-cycle variation or instability in amplitude |
| Sjogren's syndrome | chronic inflammatory autoimmune disease which results in dryness of mucous membranes (especially eyes and mouth) |
| Stephens-Johnson syndrome | a severe autoimmune disorder causing erythema and inflammation of mucous membranes |
| strained-strangled | perceived strain or pushed vocal quality at the onset of and in maintaining phonation |
| stridor | often called *noisy breathing*; noise on inspiration as heard during ingressive phonation (Stridor warrants further medical evaluation as it may indicate an upper airway narrowing or obstruction.) |
| subglottic | below the glottis |
| superior | from above |
| supraglottic | above the glottis |
| symmetry | the degree that the vocal folds provide mirror images of one another |
| thyroplasty | a surgical procedure in which a silicone wedge is placed in the thyroid cartilage to "push" the vocal fold into midline |
| tidal volume (TV) | the volume of air inspired and expired (moved) during a typical resting respiratory cycle (750cc) |
| total glossectomy | complete surgical resection of the tongue |
| tracheomalacia | collapse of the walls of the trachea caused by soft or weakened cartilage |
| tremor | inability to produce a steady sustained tone; regular and rhythmic variations in pitch and loudness that are not under voluntary control (usually of a central nervous system [CNS] origin) |
| trismus | spasm of the muscles associated with mastication |
| vital capacity (VC) | the total volume of air that can expired after maximal inhalation (3500-5000cc for normal healthy males); VC is affected by height, weight, and age. |
| vocal fatigue | reported complaint of "tired of talking"; the need to use increased effort to talk, especially after a period of prolonged voice use |
| whisper | complete breathiness; increased airflow through slightly abducted vocal folds |

# RESOURCES

## Manufacturers and Distributors

### ACOUSTIC ANALYSIS

Kay Elemetrics Corp.
2 Bridgewater Lane
Lincoln Park, NJ 07035
973-628-6200
973-628-6363 (fax)
info@kayelemetrics.com
www.kayelemetrics.com

Tiger DRS Inc.
PO Box 75063
Seattle, WA 98125
206-499-5757
206-367-2672 (fax)
tiger-electronics@worldnet.att.net
www.drspeech.com

### AERODYNAMIC ASSESSMENT

Kay Elemetrics Corp.
2 Bridgewater Lane
Lincoln Park, NJ 07035
973-628-6200
973-628-6363 (fax)
info@kayelemetrics.com
www.kayelemetrics.com

Nagashima (Manufacturer)
Kelleher Medical, Inc. (Distributor)
2824 Anwell Drive
Richmond, VA 23235-3112
804-323-4040
804-323-4073 (fax)
kellmed@kelehermedical.com
www.kellehermedical.com

### CLASSROOM AMPLIFICATION

Sennheiser Electronic Corporation
1 Enterprise Drive
Old Lyme, CT 06371
860-434-9190
860-434-1759 (fax)
www.sennheiserusa.com

Williams Sound
TeachLogic, Inc. (distributor)
22981 Triton Way
Suite C
Laguna Hills, CA 92653
949-951-6822
800-588-0018
www.teachlogic.com

Audio Enhancement
14241 South Redwood Road
P.O. Box 2000
Bluffdale, UT 84065
801-254-9263
800-383-9362
801-254-3802 (fax)
www.audioenhancement.com

Telex Communications, Inc.
12000 Portland Avenue South
Burnsville, MN 55337
800-328-3102
866-292-7707 (fax)
www.telex.com/hearing

### EDUCATIONAL SOFTWARE

Blue Tree Publishing
8927 192nd Street SW
Edmonds, WA 98026
425-210-4743
425-697-7155 (fax)
www.bluetreepublishing.com

## LARYNGECTOMY

Atos Medical Inc.
2202 N. Bartlett Avenue
Milwaukee, WI 53202-1009
414-227-3675 (800-217-0025)
414-227-9033 (fax)
www.atosmedical.com

Boston Medical Products
117 Flanders Road
Westborough, MA 01581
508-898-9300 (800-433-2674)
508-898-2373 (fax)
www.bosmed.com

Bruce Medical Supply
411 Waverly Oaks Road, Suite 154
Waltham, MA 02452
800-225-8446
781-894-9519 (fax)
sales@brucemedical.com
www.brucemedical.com

Communicative Medical, Inc.
P.O. Box 8241
Spokane, WA 99203-0241
509-838-1060 (800-944-6801)
509-838-3948 (fax)
www.communicativemedical.com

Inhealth Technologies
1110 Mark Avenue
Carpinteria, CA 93013-2918
805-684-9337 (800-477-5969)
805-684-8594 (888-371-1530) fax
info@inhealth.com
www.inhealth.com

Lauder Enterprises
P.O. Box 780249
San Antonio, TX 78278-0249
800-388-8642
210-492-1584 (fax)
info@voicestore.com
www.voicestore.com

Luminaud Inc.
8688 Tyler Boulevard
Mentor, OH 44060
440-255-9082 (800-255-3408)
440-255-2250 (fax)
info@luminaud.com
www.luminaud.com

Portex Inc. (formerly Bivona)
10 Bowman Drive
Keene, NH 03431
www.portex.com

Professional Speech Aid Service
20 Hartford Road, Suite 30
Salem, CT 06420
863-859-2807 (800-454-7778)
info@speechaid.com
www.speechaid.com

## VIDEOSTROBOSCOPY

JedMed Instrumentation
5416 JEDMED Court
St. Louis, MO 63129-2221
314-845-3770
314-845-3441 (fax)
JEDMED@attglobal.net
www.jedmed.com

Kay Elemetrics Corp.
2 Bridgewater Lane
Lincoln Park, NJ 07035
973-628-6200
973-628-6363 (fax)
info@kayelemetrics.com
www.kayelemetrics.com

Richard Wolf Medical Instruments Corp.
353 Corporate Woods Parkway
Vernon Hills, IL 60061
847-913-1113
847-913-1488 (fax)
www.richard-wolf.com

# Organizations and Support Groups

## AMYOTROPHIC LATERAL SCLEROSIS

Amyotrophic Lateral Sclerosis Association
27001 Agoura Road, Suite 150
Calabasus Hills, CA 91301
818-880-9007
www.alsa.org

## HUNTINGTON DISEASE

158 West 29th Street
7th Floor
New York, NY 10001-5300
800-345-HDSA
212-239-3430 (fax)
www.hdsa.org

## LARYNGECTOMY

American Cancer Society
800-ACS-2345
www.cancer.org

Information Hotline for Laryngectomees and
Head/Neck Cancer Patients
Head and Neck Cancer Rehabilitation Institute
7440 North Shadeland Avenue, Suite 100
Indianapolis, IN 46250
800-305-0117

International Association of Laryngectomees
8900 Thorton Road
Box 99311
Stockton, CA 95209
866-425-3678
209-472-0516 (fax)
IAL@larynxlink.com
www.larynxlink.com

National Cancer Institute
NCI Public Inquiries Office
Suite 3036A
6116 Executive Boulevard., MSC8322
Bethesda, MD 20892-8322
1-800-422-6237
www.cancer.gov

Organization of Women Laryngectomy Survivors
877-4200WLS
info@oowls.org
www.oowls.org

The Cancer Information Network
221-227 Canal Street, Suite 409
New York, NY 10013
www.cancerlinksusa.com/larynx/

Webwhispers
www.webwhispers.org

## MYASTHENIA GRAVIS

Myasthenia Gravis Foundation of America
5841 Cedar Lake Road, Suite 204
Minneapolis, MN 55416
952-545-9438 (800-541-5454)
952-545-6073 (fax)
www.myasthenia.org

## PARKINSON'S DISEASE

American Parkinson Disease Association
1250 Hylan Boulevard, Suite 4B
Staten Island, NY 10305-1946
800-223-2732
718-981-4399 (fax)
www.apdaparkinson.com

National Parkinson Foundation, Inc.
Bob Hope Parkinson Research Center
1501 N.W. 9th Avenue
Bob Hope Road
Miami, FL 33136-1494
305-547-6666 (800-327-4545)
305-243-4403 (fax)
Claudia Espinoza, Support Group Coordinator
800-327-4545 X2985
espinoza@parkinson.org
www.Parkinson.org

Parkinson's Disease Foundation
William Black Medical Building
Columbia-Presbyterian Medical Center
710 West 168th St
www.parkinsons-foundation.org
New York, NY 10032-9982
212-923-4700 (800-457-6676)
212-923-4778 (fax)

United Parkinson Foundation
833 West Washington Boulevard
Chicago, IL 60607
313-733-1893
upfitf@msn.com

## PROGRESSIVE SUPRANUCLEAR PALSY

Society for Progressive Supranuclear Palsy
Woodholme Medical Building, Suite 515
1838 Greene Tree Road
Baltimore, MD 21208
410-486-3330 (800-457-4777)
410-486-4283 (fax)
spsp@psp.org
www.psp.org

## SPASMODIC DYSPHONIA

National Spasmodic Dysphonia Association
East Wacker Drive, Suite 2430
Chicago, IL 60601-1905
800-795-NSDA
312-803-0138 (fax)
NSDA@dysphonia.org
www.dysphonia.org

# REFERENCES

American Speech-Language-Hearing Association. (2005). *The use of voice therapy in the treatment of dysphonia* [Technical Report]. Available from www.asha.org/policy

American Speech-Language-Hearing Association. (2004). *Knowledge and skills for speech-language pathologists with respect to vocal tract visualization and imaging* [Knowledge and Skills]. Available from www.asha.org/policy

American Speech-Language-Hearing Association. (2004). *Vocal tract visualization and imaging* [Position Statement]. Available from www.asha.org/policy

American Speech-Language-Hearing Association. (2004). *Vocal tract visualization and imaging* [Technical Report]. Available from www.asha.org/policy

American Speech-Language-Hearing Association. (1998). The roles of otolaryngologists and speech-language pathologists in the performance and interpretation of strobovideolaryngoscopy. *ASHA, 4* (Suppl. 18), 32.

Aminoff, M. J., Dedo, H. H., & Izdebski, K. (1978). Clinical aspects of spasmodic dysphonia. *Journal of Neurosurgery and Psychiatry, 29*, 219-233.

Andrews, G. & Ingham, R. (1971). Stuttering: Considerations in the evaluation and treatment. *British Journal of Communication Disorders, 6*, 129-138.

Aronson, M. (1990). *Clinical voice disorders*. New York: Thieme-Stratton.

Baken, R. (1987). *Clinical management of speech and voice*. San Diego: College Hill Press.

Baken, R. & Orlokoff, R. (1999). *Clinical measurement of speech and voice* (2nd ed.). San Diego: Singular Publishing.

Bassich, C. & Ludlow, C. (1986). The use of perceptual methods by new clinicians for assessing vocal quality. *Journal of Speech and Hearing Disorder, 51*, 125-133.

Blalock, D. (1997). Speech rehabilitation after treatment of laryngeal carcinoma. *Otolaryngologic Clinics of North America, 30*, 2.

Bless, D., Hirano, M., & Feder, R. (1987). Videostroboscopic evaluation of the larynx. *Ear, Nose and Throat Journal, 66*, 289-296.

Blitzer, A. & Brin, M. F. (1992). The dystonic larynx. *Journal of Voice, 6*, 294-297.

Blom E. & Hamaker R. (1996). Chapter 42: Tracheoesophageal voice restoration following total laryngectomy. In E. N. Myers & J. Suen (Eds.), *Cancer of the head and neck*. Philadelphia: W. B. Saunders.

Boone, D. & McFarlane, S. (2000). *The voice and voice therapy* (6th ed.). Needham Heights, MA: Allyn and Bacon.

Brown, W., Vinson, B., & Crary, M. (1996). *Organic voice disorders: Assessment and treatment*. San Diego, CA: Singular Publishing.

Casper, J. & Colton, R. (1993). *Clinical manual for laryngectomy and head and neck cancer rehabilitation*. San Diego, CA: Singular Publishing.

Casper, J. & Murry, T. (2000). Voice therapy methods in dysphonia. *Otolaryngologic Clinics of North America, 33*, 5.

Colton, R. H. & Casper, J. K. (1996). *Understanding voice problems: A physiologic perspective for diagnosis and treatment* (2nd ed.). Baltimore: Lippincott, Williams & Wilkins.

Dedo, H. (1976). Recurrent laryngeal nerve section for spastic dysphonia. *Annuls of Otolaryngology, 85*, 451.

Dedo, H. H., Townsend, J. L., & Izdebski, K. (1978). Current evidence for the organic etiology of spastic dysphonia. *Otology, Rhinology & Laryngology, 86*, 875-880.

Dirckx, J. H. (Ed.). (2001). *Stedman's concise medical dictionary for the health professional* (4th ed.). Baltimore: Lippincott, Williams & Wilkins.

Duffy, J. (1995). *Motor speech disorders: Substrates, differential diagnosis, and management.* St. Louis: Mosby.

Dworkin, J. & Meleca, R. (1997). *Vocal pathologies: Diagnosis, treatment, and case studies.* San Diego, CA: Singular Publishing.

Eckel, F. & Boone, D. (1981). The s/z ratio as an indicator of laryngeal pathology. *Journal of Speech and Hearing Disorders, 46*, 147-149.

Emerich, K. & Sapir, S. (1999, November). *Voice problems in young singers: Epidemiology, causes, diagnosis and treatment.* Presented at the ASHA Convention, San Francisco, CA.

Haynes,W., Pindzola, R., & Lon L. (1992). *Diagnosis and evaluation in speech pathology* (4th ed.). Englewood Cliffs, NJ: Prentice Hall.

Higgins, M., Netsell, R., & Schulte, L. (1994). Aerodynamic and electrogtottalgraphic measures of normal voice production: Intrasubject variability within and across sessions. *Journal of Speech and Hearing Research, 37*, 38-45.

Hirano, M. (1981). Structure of the vocal fold in normal and disease states: anatomical and physiological studies. In C. Ludlow & M. Hart (Eds.), *Proceedings of the conference on assessment of vocal pathology*, (pp. 11-30). Rockville, MD: American Speech-Language-Hearing Association.

Hirano, M. & Bless, D. (1993). *Videostroboscopic examination of the larynx.* San Diego: Singular Publishing.

Hollien, H. & Shipp, T. (1972). Speaking fundamental frequency and chronological age in males. *Journal of Speech and Hearing Research, 15*, 155-159.

Holmberg, E., Hillman, R., Perkell, J., & Gress, C. (1994). Relationships between intraspeaker variation in aerodynamic measures of voice production and variation in SPL across repeated recordings. *Journal of Speech and Hearing Research, 37*, 484-495.

Karnell, M., Melton, S., Childes, J., Coleman, T., Dailey, S., & Hoffman, H. (2007). Reliability of clinician-based (GRBAS and CAPE-V) and patient-based (VRQOL and IPVI) documentation of voice disorders. *Journal of Voice, 21*(5), 576-590.

Keith, R. & Darley, F. (1994). *Laryngectomee rehabilitation* (3rd ed.). Austin, TX: Pro-Ed.

Kent, R. & Ball, M. (2000). *Voice quality measurement.* San Diego, CA: Singular Publishing.

Koufman, J. (1991). The otolaryngologic manifestations of gastroesophageal reflux disease (GERD): A clinical investigation of 225 patients using ambulatory 24-hour pH monitoring and an experimental investigation of the role of acid and pepsin in the development of laryngeal injury. *Laryngoscope, 101*, 1-78.

Koufman, J. & Blalock, D. (1991). Functional voice disorders. *Otolaryngologic Clinics of North America, 24*, 5.

Koufman, J. & Block, C. (2008). Differential diagnosis of paradoxical vocal fold movement. *American Journal Speech Language Pathology, 17*(4), 327-334.

Koufman, J. A. & Cummins, M. M. (1995, April). *The prevalence and spectrum of reflux in laryngology: A prospective study of 132 consecutive patients with laryngeal and voice disorders*. Paper presented at the annual meeting of the Triologiocal Society, Palm Springs, CA.

Koufman, J., Sataloff, R., & Toohill, R. (1996). Laryngopharyngeal reflux: Consensus conference report. *Journal of Voice, 10*, 215-216.

Kreiman, J., Gerratt, B., & Pecoda, K. (1990). Listener experience and perception of vocal quality. *Journal of Speech and Hearing Research, 33*, 103-115.

Kreiman, J., Gerratt, B., Pecoda, K., & Berke, G. (1992). Individual differences in voice quality perception. *Journal of Speech and Hearing Research, 35*, 512-520.

Lessac, A. (1997). *The use and training of the human voice: A biodynamic approach to vocal life*. Mountain View, CA: Mayfield Publishing.

Levine, P., Brasnu, D., Ruparelia, A., & Laccourreye, O. (1997). Management of advanced stage laryngeal cancer. *The Otolaryngologic Clinics of North America, 30*, 1.

Logemann, J. (1998). *Evaluation and treatment of swallowing disorders* (2nd ed.). Austin, TX: Pro-Ed.

Lowell, S., Barkmeier-Kraemer, J., Hoit, J., & Story, B. (2008). Respiratory and laryngeal function during spontaneous speaking in teachers with voice disorders. *Journal of Speech, Language, and Hearing Research, 51*, 333-349.

Mathers-Schmidt, B. (2001). Paradoxical vocal fold motion: A tutorial on a complex disorder and the speech-language pathologist's role. *American Journal of Speech-Language Pathology, 10*, 111-125.

Murry, T. & Woodson, G. (1995). Combined modality treatment of spasmodic dysphonia with botulinium toxin and voice therapy. *Journal of Voice, 9*, 460-465.

National Center for Voice and Speech. (1994). The summary statement workshop on accoustic voice analysis.

Netsell, R. & Hixon, T. (1978). A noninvasive method for clinically estimating subglottal air pressure. *Journal of Speech and Hearing Disorders, 43*, 326-330.

Pannbacker, M. (1998). Voice treatment techniques: A review and recommendations for outcome studies. *American Journal of Speech Language Pathology, 7*, 49-64.

Peters, T. & Guitar, B. (1991). *Stuttering: An integrated approach to its nature and treatment*. Baltimore, MD: Williams & Wilkin.

Prater, R. & Swift, R. (1984). *Manual of voice treatment*. Boston: Little, Brown and Company.

Ramig, L. (1995). Speech therapy for patients with Parkinson's disease. In W. C. Koller & G. Paulson (Eds.). *Therapy for Parkinson's disease* (pp. 539-550). New York: Marcel Dekker.

Ramig, L., Bonitati, C., Lemke, J., & Horii, Y. (1994). Voice treatment for patients with Parkinson's disease: Development of an approach and preliminary efficacy data. *Journal of Medical Speech Language Pathology, 2*, 191-209.

Ramig, L. & Verdolini, K. (1998). Treatment efficacy: Voice disorders. *Journal of Speech and Hearing Research, 41*, 101-116.

Rosen, C. & Murry, T. (2000). Nomenclature of voice disorders and vocal pathology. *Otolaryngologic Clinics of North America, 33*, 5, 1035-1045.

Rosen, C., Lee, A., Osborne, J., Zullo, T. & Murry, T. (2004). Development and validation of the voice handicap index-10. *Laryngoscope, 114*(9), 1549-56.

Roy, N., Merrill, R., Thibeault, S., Parsa, R., Gray, S., & Smith, M. (2004). Prevalence of voice disorders in teachers and the general population. *Journal of Speech, Language, and Hearing Research, 47*, 281-293.

Sandage, M. & Zelazny, S. (2004). Paradoxical vocal fold motion in children and adolescents. *Language, Speech, and Hearing Services in Schools, 35*, 353-362.

Sataloff, R., Mandel, S., & Rosen, D. (1997). Neurologic disorders affecting the voice in performance. In R. Sataloff (Ed.), *Professional voice: The science and art of clinical care* (2nd ed.), 42, 479-498.

Sataloff, R., Spiegel, R., Carroll, L., Schiebel, B., Darby, K., & Rulnick, R. (1988). Strobovideolaryngoscopy in professional voice users: Results and clinical value. *Journal of Voice, 1*, 359-364.

Shaw, G. & Searl, J. (1997). Laryngeal manifestations of gastroesophageal reflux before and after treatment with omeprazole. *Southern Medical Journal, 90*, 11115-1122.

Shaw, G., Searl, J., Young, J., & Miner, P. (1996). Subjective, laryngoscopic, and acoustic measurements of laryngeal reflux before and after treatment with omeprazole. *Journal of Voice, 10*, 410-418.

Smitheran, J. & Hixon, T. (1981). A clinical method for estimating laryngeal airway resistance during vowel production. *Journal of Speech and Hearing Disorders, 46*, 138-146.

Stemple, J. (1993). *Voice therapy: Clinical studies.* St. Louis, MO: Mosby Year Books.

Suntharalingam, M., Haas, M. L., Van Echo, D. A., Haddad, R., Jacobs, M. C., Levy, S., Gray, W. C., Ord, R. A., & Conley, B. A. (2001). Predictors of response and survival after concurrent chemotherapy and radiation for locally advanced squamous cell carcinomas of the head and neck. *Cancer, 91*, 548-554.

Titze, I. (1994). *Principles of voice production.* Englewood Cliffs, NJ: Prentice-Hall.

Titze, I. (1995). *Workshop on acoustic voice analysis* (Summary statement). Iowa City, IA: National Center for Voice and Speech.

Toohill, R. & Kuhn, J. (1997). Role of refluxed acid in the pathogenesis of laryngeal disorders. *American Journal of Medicine, 100*, 100S-106S.

Van den Berg, J. (1958). Myoelastic-aerodynamic theory of voice production. *Journal of Speech and Hearing Research, 1*, 227-244.

Wilson, D. (1987). *Voice problems of children* (3rd ed.). Baltimore: Williams and Wilkins.

Woo, P., Colton, R., Casper, J., & Brewer, D. (1991). Diagnostic value of stroboscopic examination in hoarse patients. *Journal of Voice, 5*(3), 231-238.

Zemlin, W. R. (1988). *Speech and hearing science: Anatomy and physiology* (3rd ed.). Englewood Cliffs, NJ: Prentice-Hall.

23-13-9